METHODS IN MOLECULAR BIOLOGY

Series Editor
John M. Walker
School of Life and Medical Sciences
University of Hertfordshire
Hatfield, Hertfordshire, AL10 9AB, UK

For further volumes:
http://www.springer.com/series/7651

Transcriptome Data Analysis

Methods and Protocols

Edited by

Yejun Wang

Department of Cell Biology and Genetics, School of Basic Medicine, Shenzhen University Health Science Center, Shenzhen, China

Ming-an Sun

Epigenomics and Computational Biology Lab, Biocomplexity Institute of Virginia Tech, Blacksburg, VA, USA

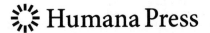

Editors
Yejun Wang
Department of Cell Biology and
Genetics, School of Basic Medicine
Shenzhen University Health
Science Center
Shenzhen, China

Ming-an Sun
Epigenomics and Computational Biology Lab
Biocomplexity Institute of Virginia Tech
Blacksburg, VA, USA

ISSN 1064-3745   ISSN 1940-6029   (electronic)
Methods in Molecular Biology
ISBN 978-1-4939-9264-5   ISBN 978-1-4939-7710-9   (eBook)
https://doi.org/10.1007/978-1-4939-7710-9

This Humana Press imprint is published by Springer Nature
The registered company is Springer Science+Business Media, LLC
The registered company address is: 233 Spring Street, New York, NY 10013, U.S.A.

Preface

As sequencing technology improves and costs decrease, more and more laboratories are performing RNA-Seq to explore the molecular mechanisms of various biological phenotypes. Due to the increased sequencing depth available, the purposes of transcriptome studies have also been expanded extensively. In addition to the conventional uses for gene annotation, profiling, and expression comparison, transcriptome studies have been applied for multiple other purposes, including but not limited to gene structure analysis, identification of new genes or regulatory RNAs, RNA editing analysis, co-expression or regulatory network analysis, biomarker discovery, development-associated imprinting studies, single-cell RNA sequencing studies, and pathogen–host dual RNA sequencing studies.

The aim of this book is to give comprehensive practical guidance on transcriptome data analysis with different scientific purposes. It is organized in three parts. In Part I, Chapters 1 and 2 introduce step-by-step protocols for RNA-Seq and microarray data analysis, respectively. Chapter 3 focuses on downstream pathway and network analysis on the differentially expressed genes identified from expression profiling data. Unlike most of the other protocols, which were command line-based, Chapter 4 describes a visualizing method for transcriptome data analysis. Chapters 5–11 in Part II give practical protocols for gene characterization analysis with RNA-Seq data, including alternative spliced isoform analysis (Chapter 5), transcript structure analysis (Chapter 6), RNA editing (Chapter 7), and identification and downstream data analysis of microRNA (Chapters 8 and 9), lincRNA (Chapter 10), and transposable elements (Chapter 11). In Part III, protocols on several new applications of transcriptome studies are described: RNA–protein interactions (Chapter 12), expression noise analysis (Chapter 13), epigenetic imprinting (Chapter 14), single-cell RNA sequencing applications (Chapter 15), and deconvolution of heterogeneous cells (Chapter 16). Some chapters cover more than one application. For example, Chapter 5 also presents the analysis of single molecule sequencing data in addition to alternative splicing analysis; Chapter 12 also gives solutions for the analysis of small RNAs in bacteria. Some topics were not included in this volume due to various factors, e.g., analysis on circular RNAs, metatranscriptomics, biomarker identification, and dual RNA-Seq. For circular RNAs, there are numerous published papers or books with protocols that can be followed. Metatranscriptomics is a new technique and data-oriented methods for analysis are still lacking. For most other applications, the core protocols for data processing and analysis are the same as presented in the chapters of this volume.

Shenzhen, China   *Yejun Wang*
Blacksburg, VA, USA   *Ming-an Sun*

Contents

Preface . . . . *v*

Contributors. . . . . *ix*

PART I   GENERAL PROTOCOLS ON TRANSCRIPTOME DATA ANALYSIS

1   Comparison of Gene Expression Profiles in Nonmodel
    Eukaryotic Organisms with RNA-Seq   3
    Han Cheng, Yejun Wang, and Ming-an Sun

2   Microarray Data Analysis for Transcriptome Profiling.   17
    Ming-an Sun, Xiaojian Shao, and Yejun Wang

3   Pathway and Network Analysis of Differentially Expressed
    Genes in Transcriptomes.   35
    Qianli Huang, Ming-an Sun, and Ping Yan

4   QuickRNASeq: Guide for Pipeline Implementation
    and for Interactive Results Visualization   57
    Wen He, Shanrong Zhao, Chi Zhang, Michael S. Vincent,
    and Baohong Zhang

PART II   OBJECTIVE-SPECIALIZED TRANSCRIPTOME DATA ANALYSIS

5   Tracking Alternatively Spliced Isoforms from Long Reads
    by SpliceHunter   73
    Zheng Kuang and Stefan Canzar

6   RNA-Seq-Based Transcript Structure Analysis with TrBorderExt   89
    Yejun Wang, Ming-an Sun, and Aaron P. White

7   Analysis of RNA Editing Sites from RNA-Seq Data Using GIREMI.   101
    Qing Zhang

8   Bioinformatic Analysis of MicroRNA Sequencing Data   109
    Xiaonan Fu and Daoyuan Dong

9   Microarray-Based MicroRNA Expression Data Analysis
    with Bioconductor   127
    Emilio Mastriani, Rihong Zhai, and Songling Zhu

10 Identification and Expression Analysis of Long Intergenic
    Noncoding RNAs.   139
    Ming-an Sun, Rihong Zhai, Qing Zhang, and Yejun Wang

11 Analysis of RNA-Seq Data Using TEtranscripts.   153
    Ying Jin and Molly Hammell

PART III   NEW APPLICATIONS OF TRANSCRIPTOME

12   Computational Analysis of RNA–Protein Interactions
     via Deep Sequencing 171
     Lei Li, Konrad U. Förstner, and Yanjie Chao

13   Predicting Gene Expression Noise from Gene Expression Variations 183
     Xiaojian Shao and Ming-an Sun

14   A Protocol for Epigenetic Imprinting Analysis with RNA-Seq Data 199
     Jinfeng Zou, Daoquan Xiang, Raju Datla, and Edwin Wang

15   Single-Cell Transcriptome Analysis Using SINCERA Pipeline 209
     Minzhe Guo and Yan Xu

16   Mathematical Modeling and Deconvolution of Molecular
     Heterogeneity Identifies Novel Subpopulations in Complex Tissues.......... 223
     Niya Wang, Lulu Chen, and Yue Wang

Index *237*

Contributors

STEFAN CANZAR • *Gene Center, Ludwig-Maximilians-Universität München, Munich, Germany*

YANJIE CHAO • *Institute of Molecular Infection Biology, University of Würzburg, Würzburg, Germany; Department of Molecular Biology and Microbiology, Howard Hughes Medical Institute, Tufts University School of Medicine, Boston, MA, USA*

LULU CHEN • *Department of Electrical and Computer Engineering, Virginia Polytechnic Institute and State University, Arlington, VA, USA*

HAN CHENG • *Key Laboratory of Rubber Biology, Ministry of Agriculture, Rubber Research Institute, Chinese Academy of Tropical Agricultural Sciences, Danzhou, Hainan, P.R. China*

RAJU DATLA • *National Research Council Canada, Saskatoon, SK, Canada*

DAOYUAN DONG • *Department of Chemistry and Biochemistry, University of the Sciences, Philadelphia, PA, USA*

KONRAD U. FÖRSTNER • *Institute of Molecular Infection Biology, University of Würzburg, Würzburg, Germany*

XIAONAN FU • *Department of Biochemistry, Virginia Tech, Blacksburg, VA, USA*

MINZHE GUO • *The Perinatal Institute, Section of Neonatology, Perinatal and Pulmonary Biology, Cincinnati Children's Hospital Medical Center, Cincinnati, OH, USA*

MOLLY HAMMELL • *Cold Spring Harbor Laboratory, Cold Spring Harbor, NY, USA*

WEN HE • *Early Clinical Development, Pfizer Worldwide R&D, Cambridge, MA, USA*

QIANLI HUANG • *School of Biological and Medical Engineering, Hefei University of Technology, Hefei, China*

YING JIN • *Cold Spring Harbor Laboratory, Cold Spring Harbor, NY, USA*

ZHENG KUANG • *Department of Immunology, The University of Texas Southwestern Medical Center, Dallas, Texas, USA*

LEI LI • *Institute of Molecular Infection Biology, University of Würzburg, Würzburg, Germany; Division of Biostatistics, Dan L. Duncan Cancer Center, Baylor College of Medicine, Houston, TX, USA*

EMILIO MASTRIANI • *Systemomics Center, College of Pharmacy, Harbin Medical University, Harbin, China; Genomics Research Center (State-Province Key Laboratories of Biomedicine-Pharmaceutics of China), Harbin Medical University, Harbin, China*

XIAOJIAN SHAO • *Department of Human Genetics, McGill University, Montréal, Canada; The McGill University and Génome Québec Innovation Centre, Montréal, QC, Canada*

MING-AN SUN • *Epigenomics and Computational Biology Lab, Biocomplexity Institute of Virginia Tech, Blacksburg, VA, USA*

MICHAEL S. VINCENT • *Inflammation and Immunology Research Unit, Pfizer Worldwide R&D, Cambridge, MA, USA*

EDWIN WANG • *Department of Experimental Medicine, McGill University, Montreal, QC, Canada; Center for Bioinformatics, McGill University, Montreal, QC, Canada; Center for Health Genomics and Informatics, University of Calgary Cumming School of Medicine, Calgary, AB, Canada; Department of Biochemistry and Molecular Biology, University of Calgary Cumming School of Medicine, Calgary, AB, Canada; Department of Medical Genetics, University of Calgary Cumming*

School of Medicine, Calgary, AB, Canada; Department of Oncology, University of Calgary Cumming School of Medicine, Calgary, AB, Canada; Alberta Children's Hospital Research Institute, Calgary, AB, Canada; Arnie Charbonneau Cancer Research Institute, Calgary, AB, Canada; O'Brien Institute for Public Health, Calgary, AB, Canada; Wang Lab, Health Science Centre, University of Calgary, Calgary, AB, Canada

NIYA WANG • *Department of Electrical and Computer Engineering, Virginia Polytechnic Institute and State University, Arlington, VA, USA*

YEJUN WANG • *Department of Cell Biology and Genetics, School of Basic Medicine, Shenzhen University Health Science Center, Shenzhen, PR China*

YUE WANG • *Department of Electrical and Computer Engineering, Virginia Polytechnic Institute and State University, Arlington, VA, USA*

AARON P. WHITE • *Vaccine and Infectious Disease Organization, University of Saskatchewan, Saskatoon, SK, Canada*

DAOQUAN XIANG • *National Research Council Canada, Saskatoon, SK, Canada*

YAN XU • *The Perinatal Institute, Section of Neonatology, Perinatal and Pulmonary Biology, Cincinnati Children's Hospital Medical Center, Cincinnati, OH, USA; Division of Biomedical Informatics, Cincinnati Children's Hospital Medical Center, Cincinnati, OH, USA*

PING YAN • *School of Biological and Medical Engineering, Hefei University of Technology, Hefei, China*

RIHONG ZHAI • *School of Public Health, Shenzhen University Health Science Center, Shenzhen, China*

BAOHONG ZHANG • *Early Clinical Development, Pfizer Worldwide R&D, Cambridge, MA, USA*

CHI ZHANG • *Early Clinical Development, Pfizer Worldwide R&D, Cambridge, MA, USA*

QING ZHANG • *Integrative Biology and Physiology, The University of California, Los Angeles (UCLA), Los Angeles, CA, USA*

SHANRONG ZHAO • *Early Clinical Development, Pfizer Worldwide R&D, Cambridge, MA, USA*

SONGLING ZHU • *Systemomics Center, College of Pharmacy, Harbin Medical University, Harbin, China; Genomics Research Center (State-Province Key Laboratories of Biomedicine-Pharmaceutics of China), Harbin Medical University, Harbin, China*

JINFENG ZOU • *National Research Council Canada, Montreal, QC, Canada*

Part I

General Protocols on Transcriptome Data Analysis

Chapter 1

Comparison of Gene Expression Profiles in Nonmodel Eukaryotic Organisms with RNA-Seq

Han Cheng, Yejun Wang, and Ming-an Sun

Abstract

With recent advances of next-generation sequencing technology, RNA-Sequencing (RNA-Seq) has emerged as a powerful approach for the transcriptomic profiling. RNA-Seq has been used in almost every field of biological studies, and has greatly extended our view of transcriptomic complexity in different species. In particular, for nonmodel organisms which are usually without high-quality reference genomes, the de novo transcriptome assembly from RNA-Seq data provides a solution for their comparative transcriptomic study. In this chapter, we focus on the comparative transcriptomic analysis of nonmodel organisms. Two analysis strategies (without or with reference genome) are described step-by-step, with the differentially expressed genes explored.

Key words Nonmodel organism, RNA-Seq, Next-generation sequencing, Differential expression, Transcriptome, de novo transcriptome assembly

1 Introduction

Recent advantages in next-generation sequencing have enabled the development of RNA-Seq—a powerful approach allowing the investigation of transcriptome at unsurpassed resolution [1]. RNA-Seq has the potential to reveal unprecedented complexity of the transcriptomes, to provide quick insights into the gene structure without the requirement of reference genome, to expand the identification for the genes of interest, to develop functional molecular markers, to quantify gene expression, and to compare gene expression profiles [2]. These advantages have made RNA-Seq the most popular method for transcriptome analysis [3]. In particular, unlike microarray which is another popular method for transcriptome profiling but needs to be designed according to presequenced reference genome, RNA-Seq could be applied for the transcriptomic study in nonmodel organisms [4]. Next-generation sequencing becomes more affordable in recent years, making RNA-Seq more and more popular in ordinary molecular biology laboratory.

Yejun Wang and Ming-an Sun (eds.), *Transcriptome Data Analysis: Methods and Protocols*, Methods in Molecular Biology, vol. 1751, https://doi.org/10.1007/978-1-4939-7710-9_1, © Springer Science+Business Media, LLC 2018

RNA-Seq has already been used in almost every field of biological studies, and has greatly extended our view of transcriptomic complexity in different species. However, the huge amounts of reads generated by RNA-Seq pose great challenges to the assembly and analysis of complete transcriptomes. Fortunately, recent progresses in bioinformatics provided powerful tools for RNA-Seq analysis of species lacking high-quality reference genome.

In nonmodel organisms, de novo transcriptome assembly is the first step for constructing a reference when the complete genome sequences are absent. In recent years, several tools have been developed for de novo transcriptome assembly, such as Trinity, SOAPdenovo-Trans, and ABYSS [4–6]. These tools each have their own merits for dealing with different types of genomes. The short reads are then mapped to the reference transcriptome, and the read counts of each transcript are normalized and compared between each sample. In this step, we usually use RSEM for quantifying transcript abundances [7]. The final step is to annotate each transcript and to visualize the expression results.

The tools mentioned above greatly facilitate transcriptome assembly and promote RNA-Seq studies in the nonmodel organisms. In recent years, a great number of studies appeared to identify differentially expressed (DE) genes between specific treatments or tissues [8–13]. In this chapter, we give a step-by-step protocol to assemble a reference transcriptome and to explore DE genes from RNA-Seq data.

2 Materials

2.1 Software Packages

All the software packages need to be installed in your workstation in advance. Because most bioinformatics tools are designed for Linux operating systems, here we demonstrate each step according to 64-bit Ubuntu OS. For the convenience of running the commands in your working directory, add the folders containing your executes into your PATH environment variable so that the executes could be used directly when you type their names. To be noted, some software used in this protocol may be not the latest version. In such case, it is highly encouraged to download the latest version for use.

2.1.1 SRA Toolkit

Download the SRA toolkit [14], unpack the tarball to your destination directory (e.g., /home/your_home/soft/), and add the executables path to your PATH, type:

```
wget http://ftp-trace.ncbi.nlm.nih.gov/sra/sdk/current/sratool
kit.current-centos_linux64.tar.gz.
```

```
tar xzf –C /home/your_home/soft/ sratoolkit.current- centos_
linux64.tar.gz
```

```
export PATH=/home/your_home/soft/sratoolkit.2.7.0-
ubuntu64/bin:$PATH
```

2.1.2 FastQC

Download the FastQC package [15], unpack and add the directory to your PATH.

```
wget   http://www.bioinformatics.bbsrc.ac.uk/projects/fastqc/
fastqc_v0.10.1.zip
```

```
unzip fastqc_v0.10.1.zip –d /home/your_home/soft/
```

```
export PATH=/home/your_home/soft/FastQC:$PATH
```

2.1.3 Trinity

Download the Trinity package [4], unpack, and add the directory to your PATH.

```
wget    https://github.com/trinityrnaseq/trinityrnaseq/archive/
v2.2.0.tar.gz.
```

```
tar xzf –C /home/your_home/soft/ trinityrnaseq-2.2.0.tar.gz
```

```
export          PATH=/home/your_home/soft/trinityrnaseq-2.2.0:
$PATH
```

```
export PATH=/home/your_home/soft/trinityrnaseq-2.2.0/
util:$PATH
```

2.1.4 RSEM

Download the RSEM package [7], unpack, and add the RSEM directory to your PATH.

```
wget https://github.com/deweylab/RSEM/archive/v1.2.8.tar.gz
```

```
tar xzf –C /home/your_home/soft/ RSEM-1.2.8.tar.gz
```

```
export PATH=/home/your_home/soft/rsem-1.2.8:$PATH
```

2.1.5 R

Download R [16], unpack and then install.

```
wget https://cran.r-project.org/src/base/R-3/R-3.2.2.tar.gz
```

```
tar zxf –C /home/your_home/soft/ R-3.2.2.tar.gz
```

```
cd /home/your_home/soft/R-3.2.2
```

```
./configure ./configure --prefix=/home/your_home/bin
```

```
make
```

```
make check
```

```
make install
```

2.1.6 Bowtie2

Download Bowtie2 package [17], unpack, and then add Bowtie2 directory to your PATH.

```
wget    http://jaist.dl.sourceforge.net/project/bowtie-bio/bow
tie2/2.2.6/bowtie2-2.2.6-linux-x86_64.zip
```

```
unzip bowtie2-2.2.6-linux-x86_64.zip -d /home/your_home/
soft/
```

```
export    PATH=/home/your_home/soft/    bowtie2-2.2.6:
$PATH
```

2.1.7 Tophat
*(See **Note 1**)*

Download Tophat [18], unpack and install, and then add the directory to your PATH.

```
wget  http://ccb.jhu.edu/software/tophat/downloads/tophat-
2.0.9.Linux_x86_64.tar.gz
```

```
tar zxf tophat-2.0.9.Linux_x86_64.tar.gz
```

```
cd tophat-2.0.9.linux_x86_64
```

```
./configure --prefix=/home/your_home/soft/tophat2
```

```
make
```

```
make install
```

```
export PATH=/home/your_home/soft/tophat2:$PATH
```

2.1.8 Cufflinks

Download Cufflinks [19], unpack and then add the directory to your PATH.

```
wget http://cole-trapnell-lab.github.io/cufflinks/assets/down
loads/cufflinks-2.2.1.Linux_x86_64.tar.gz
```

```
tar xzf –C /home/your_home/soft/ cufflinks-2.2.1.Linux_x86_
64.tar.gz
```

```
export PATH=/home/your_home/soft/cufflinks-2.2.1.Linux_
x86_64:$PATH
```

2.1.9 EBSeq

EBSeq [20] is an R Bioconductor package for gene and isoform differential expression analysis of RNA-Seq data. For installation, just start R and enter:

```
source("https://bioconductor.org/biocLite.R")
```

```
biocLite("EBSeq")
```

2.1.10 DESeq

DESeq [21] is an R Bioconductor package for differential expression analysis with reads count data. To install it, start R and enter:

```
source("https://bioconductor.org/biocLite.R")
```

```
biocLite("DESeq")
```

2.2 Data Samples

Most public RNA-Seq data could be downloaded from NCBI SRA database (https://www.ncbi.nlm.nih.gov/sra) (*see* **Note 2**). In this protocol, we use RNA-Seq data set from the rubber tree. This data set includes six samples from control and cold stressed conditions with three biological replicates, which are denoted as "control" and "cold."

3 Methods

Download the RNA-Seq data from NCBI SRA database and place the files in your working directory (e.g., /home/your_name/NGS/SRA). Run the commands as demonstrated in this protocol in your working directory (*see* **Notes 3** and **4**).

3.1 RNA-Seq Data Quality Control

1. Generate FASTQ files from SRA files. To extract FASTQ files from downloaded sra files, and put them in a new folder "fq", go to your NGS data directory and type (*see* **Note 5**):

```
fastq-dump -O ./fq --split-files ./SRA/SRR*.sra
```

2. Quality controlling by fastQC (*see* **Note 6**).

```
fastqc -o ./qc -f fastq ./fq/Sample*.fastq
```

3. Remove reads of low quality (optional). In most cases, the low quality reads have been removed when the sequences were transferred from the service supplier. In this example, the FASTQ file has been filtered when submitted to the NCBI SRA database (*see* **Note 7**).

```
fastq_quality_filter -Q33 -v -q 30 -p 90 -i fq/Sample*.fastq
-o fq/Sample*.fastq
```

3.2 Gene Expression Analysis Without Reference Genome

In most cases, nonmodel organisms do not have reference genome. We therefore use no reference genome analysis strategy to compare gene expression profiles and to find DE genes. This strategy first assembles a reference transcriptome from the RNA-Seq data, and then maps the reads to the reference transcriptome and calculates gene expression. In this protocol, we use Trinity to assemble transcriptome, and then use RSEM to calculate reads counts, finally utilize two popular packages, EBSeq and DESeq, to find DE genes respectively.

1. Reference transcriptome assembly. The Trinity program [4] can assemble the reads in all the sample files into one reference transcriptome. Then the reference transcriptome can be used for gene expression analysis. For paired-end RNA-Seq with read1 (*_1.fastq) and read2 (*_2.fastq), the reference transcriptome could be assembled by typing:

```
Trinity.pl --JM 500G --seqType fq --left fq/Sample*_1.fastq --right fq/Sample*_2.fastq --output trinity_out --min_kmer_cov 5 --CPU 32
```

(*see* **Note 8**)

   Trouble shooting: In some cases, the Trinity program will stop due to short of memory when executing the "butterfly_commands". You may go to the results directory trinity_out/chrysalis/ and check if the "butterfly_commands" file exists. Then use the following commands to continue the assembly.

```
cmd_process_forker.pl -c trinity_out/chrysalis/butterfly_commands --CPU 10 --shuffle;
```

```
find trinity_out/chrysalis -name "*allProbPaths.fasta" -exec cat {} \; > trinity_out/Trinity.fasta;
```

   You will find a "Trinity.fasta" file in the output directory, which is the assembled reference transcriptome of all the reads. You can also check the reference transcriptome statistics by running the TrinityStats.pl script provided by Trinity package:

```
TrinityStats.pl trinity_out/Trinity.fasta
```

2. Gene expression quantification with RSEM. RSEM is an accurate and user-friendly tool for quantifying transcript abundances from RNA-Seq data and it does not rely on the existence of a reference genome [7]. Therefore, it is particularly useful for expression quantification with de novo transcriptome assemblies. The RSEM program includes just two scripts (*rsem-prepare-reference* and *rsem-calculate-expression*), which invokes

Bowtie [22] for read alignment. The first step is to extract and preprocess the reference sequences and then builds Bowtie indices.

```
mkdir rsem
```

```
cd rsem
```

```
mkdir tmp
```

```
extract-transcript-to-gene-map-from-trinity ../trinity_out/
Trinity.fasta tmp/unigenes.togenes
```

```
rsem-prepare-reference   --transcript-to-gene-map   tmp/
unigenes.togene ../trinity_out/Trinity.fasta tmp/unigenes
```

Then the RNA-Seq reads in each sample are aligned to the Bowtie indices and their relative abundances are calculated. The tasks are handled by the *rsem-calculate-expression* script. By default, RSEM uses the Bowtie alignment program to align reads, with parameters specifically chosen for RNA-Seq quantification. The *rsem-calculate-expression* script processes the reads in each sample. A short Bash script will be much easier to handle large amount of samples in one analysis.

```
export k
```

```
for ((k=1;k&lt;6;k+=1));do
```

```
rsem-calculate-expression  -p  24  --bowtie-chunkmbs  512
--paired-end --no-bam-output --forward-prob 0.0 fq/Sample
${k}_1.fq fq/Sample${k}_2.fq tmp/unigenes rsem/Sample${k};
```

```
done
```

The *rsem-calculate-expression* script produces two files with ". results" suffix, in which the ".gene.results" file calculate TPM and FPKM for each gene, whereas the ".transcripts.results" listed the TPM and FPKM for each transcript. The file structures are as follow:

The "Sample.genes.results" file:

gene_id	transcript_id(s)	length	effective_length	expected_count	TPM	FPKM
c0.graph_c0	c0.graph_c0_seq1	745.00	690.31	14.00	2.43	1.79
c1.graph_c0	c1.graph_c0_seq1	262.00	207.46	1.00	0.58	0.43

The "Sample.transcripts.results" file:

transcript_id	gene_id	length	effective_length	expected_count	TPM	FPKM	IsoPct
c0.graph_c0_seq1	c0.graph_c0	745	690.31	14.00	2.43	1.79	100.00
c1.graph_c0_seq1	c1.graph_c0	262	207.46	1.00	0.58	0.43	100.00

3. Differentially expressed gene identification with EBSeq. EBSeq is an R package for exploring DE genes and isoforms from RNA-Seq data, which is based on empirical Bayesian method and aims to identify DE isoforms between two or more biological samples [20]. EBSeq processes counts matrix files generated by RSEM, and calculates the expression of each gene in each sample.

RSEM provides several wrappers which could invoke EBSeq to identify differentially expressed genes. This is the easier way to use EBSeq. Merge each single counts file to generate a matrix file with the following commands:

```
rsem-generate-ngvector ../trinity_out/Trinity.fasta cov5_trinity
```

```
rsem-generate-data-matrix Sample*.genes.results >
genes.counts.matrix
```

Then use the following commands to obtain DE genes:

```
rsem-run-ebseq --ngvector cov5_trinity.ngvec genes.
counts.matrix 3,3 GeneMat.results
```

```
rsem-control-fdr GeneMat.results 0.05 GeneMat.de.txt
```

(*see* **Note 9**)

Alternatively, you can also use EBSeq in a native way for DE gene identification. In R console, type:

```
library("EBSeq")
```

```
setwd("/path/to/your/directory/rsem/")
```

```
GeneMat    <-    data.matrix(read.table(file="genes.counts.
matrix"))
```

```
NgVec <- scan(file="cov5_trinity.ngvec", what=0, sep="\n")
```

```
Condition = factor(c("Control","Control","Control","Cold",
"Cold","Cold"))
```

```
GeneSizes = MedianNorm(GeneMat)
```

```
GeneEBOut = EBTest (Data=GeneMat, Conditions=Condi-
tion,sizeFactors=GeneSizes, maxround=10)
```

```
GeneEBDERes=GetDEResults(GeneEBOut, FDR=0.05)
```

(*see* **Note 9**)

For more detailed function introduction, please refer EBSeq vignette [20].

4. Differentially expressed gene identification with DESeq. Alternatively, you can use DESeq for DE gene identification. DESeq is a R package to analyze sequence counts data from RNA-Seq and test for differential expression [21]. DESeq accepts RSEM output files for analysis. The first step is to merge each FPKM count files generated by *rsem-calculate-expression* script in RSEM package. The merging step can be performed with *merge_RSEM_frag_counts_single_table.pl* scripts from Trinity package:

```
TRINITY_HOME/util/RSEM_util/merge_RSEM_frag_
counts_single_table.pl Sample1.genes.results Sample2.genes.results
Sample3.genes.results Sample4.genes.results Sample5.genes.results
>all.genes.counts
```

Then in R console, type:

```
library("DESeq")
```

```
countTable<-read.table("all.genes.counts",header=T,sep=
"\t",row.names=1)
```

```
countTable = round(countTable)
```

(*see* **Note 10**)

```
conditions<-factor(c("Control","Control","Control",
"Cold","Cold","Cold"))
```

```
cds<-newCountDataSet(countTable,conditions)
```

```
cds<-estimateSizeFactors(cds)
```

```
cds<-estimateDispersions(cds)
```

```
res <-nbinomTest(cds,"Control","Cold") #call differential
expression
```

```
write.table(res, 'compare.csv',sep='\t',quote=F,row.names=F)
```

```
head(res)
```

```
plotMA(res)
```

```
res_sig<-subset(res, padj<0.05);
```
    (*see* **Note 11**)

```
dim(res_sig)
```

```
res_sig_order<-res_sig[order(res_sig$padj),]
```

```
write.table(res_sig_order, 'difference.txt',sep='\t',quote=F,
row.names=F)
```
    (*see* **Note 12**)

For detailed introduction, please refer to DESeq vignette [23].

3.3 Gene Expression Analysis with Reference Genome

Benefiting from genome sequencing projects, many reference genomes have been published in nonmodel organisms recently. In these organisms, the analysis strategy with reference genome can be adopted. Typically, we first prepare the reference genome files, then map each reads file to the reference genome, and finally call the DE genes.

1. Prepare reference genome file. Download the genome files (sequence fasta file and gff annotation file) from GenBank database, and then build the bowtie2 index with "*bowtie2-build*" command in Bowtie2 package:

```
bowtie2-build /path/to/genome/HbGenome.fas bowtie-ref/Hbgenome
```

(*see* **Note 13**)

2. Map reads to reference genome. Map each reads file to the genome index with *tophat2* program, and then assemble transcripts from the reads file with *cufflinks* program:

```
tophat2 -o 1th -p 32 -G /path/to/gff/HbGenome.gff3
bowtie-ref/HbGenome /path/to/sample1/Sample1_1.fq/
path/to/sample/Sample1_2.fq
```

```
cufflinks -p 32 -o 1cl 1th/accepted_hits.bam
```

You may use a short Bash script to analyze several samples in one command:

```
export k;
```

```
for ((k=1;k&lt;6;k+=1));do
```

```
tophat2 -o ${k}th -p 32 -G /path/to/gff/HbGenome.gff3
bowtie-ref/HbGenome /path/to/sample1/Sample${k}_1.fq/
path/to/sample/Sample${k}_2.fq;
```

```
cufflinks -p 32 -o ${k}cl ${k}th/accepted_hits.bam;
```

```
done
```

Then merge all the assembled transcripts files:

```
ls *cl/transcripts.gtf >assemblies.txt
```

```
cuffmerge -p 32 -g /path/to/gff/HbGenome.gff3 -s /
path/to/genome /HbGenome.fas assemblies.txt
```

(*see* **Note 14**)

3. Call differential expression genes with Cuffdiff. Cufflinks includes a program, "Cuffdiff", which can be used to find significant changes in transcript expression, splicing, and promoter use. Cuffdiff requires two types of files: sam (or bam) file from Tophat program and transcript annotation gtf file from cufflinks:

```
cuffdiff -o diff_out/ -b /path/to/genome/Hbgenome.fa
-L Control,Cold -u merged_asm/merged.gtf -p 8 1th/accep-
ted_hits.bam,2th/accepted_hits.bam,3th/accepted_hits.bam
4th/accepted_hits.bam,5th/accepted_hits.bam,6th/accepted_
hits.bam
```

(*see* **Note 15**)

The comparison results will be wrote to "diff_out" directory. Several comparison results will be found, including cds, isoform, gene, tss, splicing, and promoter. In most cases, you may be interested in "gene_exp.diff" file. Then you can extract DE genes from this file based on your criteria and the adjusted "q_value". The content of the diff file:

test_id gene_id gene locus sample_1 sample_2 status value_1 value_2 log2(fold_change) test_stat p_value q_value significant

XLOC_000001 XLOC_000001 - scaffold0001:445549-451760   Control   Cold OK 4.17386 2.62692 -0.668007   -0.799812   0.1381   0.404678   no

4   Notes

1. The *Tophat2* was superseded by *HISAT2*. In this protocol, we still use old version Tophat for analysis.

2. To simplify the analysis procedure, we use nonmodel *Hevea brasiliensis* (rubber tree) RNA-Seq data as the example. This dataset include two samples (Leaf under control condition, and cold treated for 24 h), each with three biological replicates.

3. This protocol only shows how to run each analysis steps, and also gives frequently used options for each command or scripts. You may also go to check each option of the command and optimize your own analysis parameters.

4. Please note that the directory structural differences between this protocol and your own workstation. You should change the file paths and names according to your own directory.

5. The *fastq-dump* tool extract reads from SRA package. The parameter "-O" defines the output directory. "--split-files" option will enable dumping each read into separate file. Files will receive suffix corresponding to read number.

6. The results are in the subdirectory under the name of fastq filename with a "_fastqc" suffix. You may examine the detail quality check results in "astqc_report.html" file.

7. Add the "-Q33" parameter when meet "fastq_quality_filter: Invalid quality score value" error.

8. "--JM" option defines how much Giga memory allocated for the jellyfish to calculate k-mer. --left and --right define the left and right fastq files for the pair-end seuqencing results. --min_kmer_cov defines the minimal kmer when calculate the k-mer number in Inchworm, a high --min_kmer_cov value will reduce the noise in the assembly and to identify only transcripts that were relatively highly expressed, but also lose some lowly expressed transcripts. Define --CPU number for the inchworm when your server has multiple CPU.

9. This analysis found DE genes at the target FDR of 0.05.

10. Expected_counts from RSEM are float numbers because the reads mapped to multiple locations are assigned to each location according to the fractional weighted estimation using an EM algorithm. However, the DESeq only accepts integer counts. We therefore use round function to get integer counts.

11. Get DE genes by adjusted p-value less than 0.05.

12. The scripts find DE genes by adjusted p-value less than 0.05, then export DE gene list to the "difference.txt" file.

13. The *bowtie2-build* command builds an "Hbgenome" genome index from genome file "HbGenome.fas".

14. The program will generate a "merged.gtf" file in "merged_asm" directory.

15. Supply replicate SAMs as comma separated lists for each condition: Sample1_rep1.sam,sample1_rep2.sam,...sample1_repM.sam. Separate each condition with space. -L/――labels, comma-separated list of condition labels. Each lable indict one treatment (condition); The label numbers should equal to conditions.

Acknowledgments

This work is supported by the National Natural Science Foundation of China (grant No. 31301072).

References

1. Hoeijmakers WAM, Bártfai R, Stunnenberg HG (2013) Transcriptome analysis using RNA-Seq. Methods Mol Biol 923:221–239

2. Garg R, Jain M (2013) RNA-Seq for transcriptome analysis in non-model plants. Methods Mol Biol 1069:43–58

3. Wang Z, Gerstein M, Snyder M (2009) RNA-Seq: a revolutionary tool for transcriptomics. Nat Rev Genet 10:57–63

4. Grabherr MG, Haas BJ, Yassour M et al (2011) Full-length transcriptome assembly from RNA-Seq data without a reference genome. Nat Biotechnol 29:644–652

5. Xie Y, Wu G, Tang J et al (2014) SOAPdenovo-trans: de novo transcriptome assembly with short RNA-Seq reads. Bioinformatics 30:1660–1666

6. Simpson JT, Wong K, Jackman SD et al (2009) ABySS: a parallel assembler for short read sequence data. Genome Res 19:1117–1123

7. Li B, Dewey CN (2011) RSEM: accurate transcript quantification from RNA-Seq data with or without a reference genome. BMC Bioinformatics 12:323

8. Chao J, Chen Y, Wu S, Tian W-M (2015) Comparative transcriptome analysis of latex from rubber tree clone CATAS8-79 and PR107 reveals new cues for the regulation of latex regeneration and duration of latex flow. BMC Plant Biol 15:104

9. Fang Y, Mei H, Zhou B et al (2016) De novo Transcriptome analysis reveals distinct Defense mechanisms by young and mature leaves of Hevea Brasiliensis (Para rubber tree). Sci Rep 6:33151

10. Bevilacqua CB, Basu S, Pereira A et al (2015) Analysis of stress-responsive gene expression in cultivated and weedy Rice differing in cold stress tolerance. PLoS One 10:e0132100

11. Fu J, Miao Y, Shao L et al (2016) De novo transcriptome sequencing and gene expression profiling of Elymus Nutans under cold stress. BMC Genomics 17:870

12. Nakashima K, Yamaguchi-Shinozaki K, Shinozaki K (2014) The transcriptional regulatory network in the drought response and its cross-talk in abiotic stress responses including drought, cold, and heat. Front Plant Sci 5:170

13. An D, Yang J, Zhang P (2012) Transcriptome profiling of low temperature-treated cassava apical shoots showed dynamic responses of tropical plant to cold stress. BMC Genomics 13:64

14. SRA Toolkit: https://trace.ncbi.nlm.nih.gov/Traces/sra/

15. FastQC: http://www.bioinformatics.babraham.ac.uk/projects/fastqc/

16. R: The R Project for Statistical Computing. https://www.r-project.org/

17. Langmead B, Salzberg SL (2012) Fast gapped-read alignment with bowtie 2. Nat Methods 9:357–359

18. Kim D, Pertea G, Trapnell C et al (2013) TopHat2: accurate alignment of transcriptomes in the presence of insertions, deletions and gene fusions. Genome Biol 14:R36

19. Trapnell C, Roberts A, Goff L et al (2012) Differential gene and transcript expression analysis of RNA-seq experiments with TopHat and cufflinks. Nat Protoc 7:562–578

20. Leng N, Dawson JA, Thomson JA et al (2013) EBSeq: an empirical Bayes hierarchical model for inference in RNA-seq experiments. Bioinformatics 29:1035–1043

21. Anders S, Huber W (2010) Differential expression analysis for sequence count data. Genome Biol 11:R106

22. Langmead B, Trapnell C, Pop M, Salzberg SL (2009) Ultrafast and memory-efficient alignment of short DNA sequences to the human genome. Genome Biol 10:R25

23. Love MI, Anders S, Kim V, Huber W (2015) RNA-Seq workflow: gene-level exploratory analysis and differential expression. F1000Res 4:1070

Chapter 2

Microarray Data Analysis for Transcriptome Profiling

Ming-an Sun, Xiaojian Shao, and Yejun Wang

Abstract

Microarray data have vastly accumulated in the past two decades. Due to the high-throughput characteristic of microarray techniques, it has transformed biological studies from specific genes to transcriptome level, and deeply boosted many fields of biological studies. While microarray offers great advantages for expression profiling, on the other hand it faces a lot challenges for computational analysis. In this chapter, we demonstrate how to perform standard analysis including data preprocessing, quality assessment, differential expression analysis, and general downstream analyses.

Key words Microarray, Normalization, Clustering, Differential expression, Bioconductor, Limma, GeneFilter

1 Introduction

The successful application of microarray for expression analysis could be traced back to two decades ago [1]. Since then, the microarray technique has been widely used for expression profiling in almost every field of biological research [2]. Beyond transcription analysis, alternative microarray based techniques have also been designed for other purposes such as genotyping, DNA mapping, protein binding, and epigenetic studies [3]. Due to the high-throughput characteristics of microarray techniques, it has transformed biological studies from specific genes to transcriptome level, and deeply boosted many fields of biological studies. Previous studies showed that microarray is robust for measuring transcriptome [4]. Even though RNA-Seq has emerged in recent years, microarrays remain popular for measuring gene expression [5, 6]. In particular, since microarray is cheaper than RNA-Seq, it has advantages for clinical studies, which may involve a huge amount of samples. For example, microarray is frequently used in several comprehensive projects for cancers, including The Cancer Genome Atlas project [7].

Yejun Wang and Ming-an Sun (eds.), *Transcriptome Data Analysis: Methods and Protocols*, Methods in Molecular Biology, vol. 1751, https://doi.org/10.1007/978-1-4939-7710-9_2, © Springer Science+Business Media, LLC 2018

While microarray offers great advantages for expression profiling, on the other hand it faces a lot challenges for analysis [2]. In particular, technical noise could be introduced in microarray data. Additionally, the challenges of analysis also come from the tremendous number of probes in microarray, and the few number of replicates used for most microarray studies. Currently, a large number of methods have been proposed to deal with problems for each analysis step, including quality control [8–10], normalization [11], and differential expression analysis [12–14].

Bioconductor is an open-source, open-development software project for the analysis and comprehension of high-throughput data arising from genomics and molecular biology [15]. So far more than 1000 packages have been released in the Bioconductor. Importantly, every step for microarray data analysis could find a solution using packages hosted in Bioconductor project (*see* **Note 1**). In this chapter, we show how to implement each step of microarray analysis, including quality control, normalization, differential expression analysis and some general downstream analyses, using packages mainly from Bioconductor project. In this protocol, data generated from Affymetrix Mouse Gene 2.0 ST Array (MoGene-2.0-ST) platform was used for demonstration. However, the analysis procedure described in this protocol could be adjusted for the analysis of data from other microarray platforms easily.

2   Materials

2.1   Microarray Data

This protocol starts with Affymetrix microarray data of CEL format (*see* **Note 2**). The CEL files store the results of the calculated intensity. In addition to newly generated CEL files in the lab, a huge amount of published CEL files could be retrieved from several public resources, in particular ArrayExpress (https://www.ebi.ac.uk/arrayexpress/) and NCBI Gene Expression Ominibus (GEO; https://www.ncbi.nlm.nih.gov/geo/). To be noted, ArrayExpress is specific for microarray data, while GEO also contains other types of OMICs data.

In this protocol, we use public datasets (GEO accession: GSE67964) for Affymetrix Mouse Gene 2.0 ST Array (MoGene-2.0-ST) for demonstration.

2.2   R Packages

This protocol involves a number of R packages, thus basic knowledge about R and Bioconductor is essential. The basics of R could be found from resources such as http://tryr.codeschool.com/. R and Bioconductor could be installed by following instructions from http://www.bioconductor.org/install/. Below we briefly summarized the ways for R and Bioconductor packages installation and loading (*see* **Note 3**). For the installation of each package used in this protocol, it will be described in the corresponding section.

R packages could be installed using the *install.packages()* function easily. Take ggplot2 package as example, you just need to start the R console and type:

```
install.packages("ggplot2")
```

To install core packages from Bioconductor, type:

```
source("https://bioconductor.org/biocLite.R")
```

Then, specific Bioconductor packages could be installed. For example, to install the oligo package, type:

```
biocLite("oligo")
```

After installation, both R or Bioconductor packages could be loaded by the *library()* function. Take the oligo package as example, to load it, type:

```
library(oligo)
```

2.3 Annotation Files

Two types of annotation files are required: (1) the probe set annotation, which summarizes the location of all probes on the array, as well as the probes for each probe set; (2) gene annotation, which maps the probesets to their corresponding genes.

For most microarray platforms, R Bioconductor packages providing the annotation information are ready for use (*see* **Note 1**). For example, the two annotation packages for MoGene2.0-ST microarray are pd.mogene.2.0.st [16] and mogene20sttranscriptcluster.db [17], respectively. Since this protocol involves a lot of R Bioconductor packages, these annotation packages could be incorporated into the pipeline seamlessly.

3 Methods

3.1 Data Preprocessing

We download CEL files from GEO (https://www.ncbi.nlm.nih.gov/geo/) by searching GEO accession (e.g., GSE67964). This dataset contains data for wild-type and ROR_alpha_gamma_dKO, each with four replicates.

3.1.1 Prepare Data

3.1.2 Set Work Directory

To set the work directory, type:

```
setwd("directory_with_CEL_files")
```

3.1.3 Read Data into Memory

The Bioconductor package "oligo" offers a number of tools for preprocessing of Affymetrix CEL files, including data import, background correction, normalization, data summarization and visualization [18]. In addition, you might need to install and load the probe set annotation package (e.g., pd.mogene.2.0.st for MoGene2.0-ST platform), if it is failed to be installed automatically together with "oligo".

1. To install and load the oligo package, type:

```
biocLite("oligo")
library(oligo)
```

2. To get the list of all the CEL files in the directory, type:

```
cel.files <- list.celfiles()
```

Or if you only want to read specific CEL files (e.g., celfile1 and celfile2), type:

```
cel.files <- c(celfile1, celfile2)
```

3. By default, CEL file names will be specified as sample names. However, we usually want to respecify sample names, in particular when the CEL file names are lengthy. The sample names should be of the same number and order of CEL file names. To specify sample names manually, type:

```
sample.names = c("WT1", "WT2", "WT3", "WT4","KO1", "KO2",
"KO3", "KO4")
```

4. To read CEL files into memory, type:

```
affy.raw <- read.celfiles(cel.files, sampleNames = sample.
names)
```

3.1.4 Get Normalized Gene Expression

To summarize gene level expression, the probeset annotation for specific array is required. Take microarray data from mogene.2.0.st platform as example, the Bioconductor package pd.mogene.2.0.st [16] is needed.

1. To install and load the annotation library pd.mogene.2.0.st, type:

```
biocLite("pd.mogene.2.0.st")
library(pd.mogene.2.0.st)
```

2. To make reasonable comparison between different samples, normalization must be performed. Robust Multi-Array Average (RMA) is the most widely used normalization algorithm. Meanwhile, there are several other normalization algorithms, including GCRMA, Mas5, dChip, and so on (*see* **Note 4**). The differences of these methods have been discussed in previous

studies []. The GCRMA package takes GC content into account when doing RMA normalization. However, one study argued that a crucial step in GCRMA responsible for introducing severe artifacts in the data leading to a systematic overestimate of pairwise correlation []. Here we show the use of RMA, but you could apply other your preferred algorithms. To normalize gene expression using RMA algorithm, and create an ExpressionSet object (*see* **Note 5**), type:

```
eset <- rma(affy.raw)
```

3. To save the expression data in a local file that may be used later (to be noted, the expression values in the output are normalized and log2 transformed), type:

```
write.exprs(eset,file="rma_norm_expr.txt")
```

3.1.5 Gene Annotation

Gene annotation is need for further interpretation of the results. Two Bioconductor packages are required, including Biobase [15] and mogene20sttranscriptcluster.db [17].

1. To install and load these two packages, type:

```
biocLite("Biobase")
biocLite("mogene20sttranscriptcluster.db")
library(Biobase)
library(mogene20sttranscriptcluster.db)
```

2. The mogene20sttranscriptcluster.db package provides a variety of detailed information for Mogene2.0ST platform, including ACCNUM, ENSEMBL, ENTREZID, ENZYME, GENE-NAME, GO, PATH, PFAM, PROSIT, REFSEQ, SYMBOL, UNIGENE, and UNIPROT. To get a list of available objects in the package, type:

```
keytypes(mogene20sttranscriptcluster.db)
```

3. To retrieve data for selected objects (e.g., ENTREZID and SYMBOL as showed below) as a data frame, type:

```
gns <- select(mogene20sttranscriptcluster.db, keys(mogen-
e20sttranscriptcluster.db), c("ENTREZID", "SYMBOL"))
```

4. For certain types of annotations (such as gene symbol), there could be multiple matches for the same gene. In such case, if you only want to keep one match per gene, the most naive way is to keep the first one. However, just skip this step if you want to use full annotation information. To keep only the first annotation for each gene, type:

```
gns <- gns[!duplicated(gns[,1]),]
```

5. To convert the gene annotation matrix by setting row names to probe ID (so it will be more convenient for further use), type:

```
gns = gns[,-1]
row.names(gns) = keys(mogene20sttranscriptcluster.db)
```

6. To retrieve gene expression matrix from eset as a data frame, type:

```
expr <- data.frame(exprs(eset))
```

7. To merge gene expression data and annotation data together according to row names, which are probe IDs in this case, type:

```
expr.anno <- merge(gns, expr, by.x=0, by.y=0, all=TRUE)
```

8. To save the annotated gene expression matrix to local file for further use, type:

```
write.table(expr.anno, file = "rma_norm_expr.anno.txt",
sep = "\t", row.names = FALSE, col.names = TRUE, quote =
FALSE)
```

3.2 Quality Assessment

The assessment of data quality is an essential step for microarray analysis. There are different tools and packages developed for microarray quality assessment [9, 10]. Among them, arrayQuality-Metrics [8] is a Bioconductor package that provides quality metrics to assess reproducibility, identify apparent outlier arrays, and compute measures of signal-to-noise ratio.

The arrayQualityMetrics package produces a comprehensive report of quality metrics about a microarray dataset. The quality metrics are mainly on per array level, but meanwhile, some of the metrics can also be used to diagnose batch effects. When the function *arrayQualityMetrics* is finished, a report is produced in the directory specified by the function's outdir argument.

1. To install and load arrayQualityMetrics package, type:

```
biocLite("arrayQualityMetrics")
library(arrayQualityMetrics")
```

2. The AffyBatch object affy.raw as generated in **step 4** of Subheading 3.1.3 could be used as input. To get the quality assessment results, type:

```
arrayQualityMetrics(expressionset = affy.raw, outdir =
"QC_report_for_raw", force = TRUE, do.logtransform = TRUE)
```

3. Alternatively, we can also use the preprocessed dataset (e.g., the normalized data eset we obtained previously) for quality assessment. To be noted, if the data have already been log2-scaled

after normalization (such as RMA), it is not needed to set the do.logtransform parameter now. To run *arrayQualityMetrics* using the processed data, type:

```
arrayQualityMetrics(expressionset = eset, outdir = "QC_re-
port_for_rma", force = TRUE)
```

arrayQualityMetrics will produce a folder containing all results. By opening the index.html file, you could find the results organized as "between array comparison", "array intensity distributions", "variance mean dependence" and "individual array quality".

3.3   Gene Filtering

Microarray could typically monitor the expression of tens of thousands of genes. Accordingly, a huge number of hypothesis tests are performed to detect differentially expressed genes, and many true-null hypotheses will produce small p-values by chance. As a consequence, it is necessary to further apply multiple testing adjustment to control such false positive measures, e.g., the family-wise error rate (FWER) or the false discovery rate (FDR). Nevertheless, multiple testing adjustment also reduces the power to detect true positives.

Due to the inherited noise from microarray technique, and the fact that only a small number of replicates are used in most studies, it is common that for many studies no differentially expressed genes could be detected after multiple testing adjustment. Previous studies showed that independent filtering steps could remarkably increase the power for differential gene detection from high-throughput experiments [20, 21].

Here we show how to remove probe sets with low expression and low variance across all arrays using the R package genefilter [22]. Just skip the following steps if you don't want to perform gene filtering.

1. To install and load genefilter package, type:

```
install.packages("genefilter")
library(genefilter)
```

2. To remove probe sets with low variance across all arrays (those with variance below the 0.25 quantile), and show the number after filtering, type:

```
eset.filt = varFilter(eset.filt, var.func=IQR, var.cutoff
= 0.25, filterByQuantile = TRUE)
nrow(eset.filt)
```

3. To remove probe sets without gene annotation information, and show the number after filtering, type:

```
eset.filt = eset.filt[featureNames(eset.filt) %in%
row.names(gns)[!is.na(gns$SYMBOL)], ]
nrow(eset.filt)
```

4. To remove probe sets with multiple gene symbols, and show the number after filtering, type:

```
eset.filt = eset.filt[featureNames(eset.filt) %in%
row.names(gns)[!duplicated(gns$SYMBOL)],]
nrow(eset.filt)
```

3.4 Differential Expression Analysis

One of the major purposes of using microarray is to detect differentially expressed genes between different conditions (e.g., normal vs. tumor, treatment vs. untreatment) or during time series process. The Bioconductor package limma [14] provides integrated methods for gene expression analysis, and could handle complex experimental designs. In this protocol, we show how to perform differential expression using limma. To be noted, alternative methods such as SAM [12] and RankProduct [13] are also widely used for differential analysis (*see* **Note 6**).

To install and load limma, type:

```
biocLite("limma")
library(limma)
```

3.4.1 Create Design Matrix

The first step is to create design matrix to describe the features (such as treated or untreated) for each sample. Suppose you want to compare the gene expression between wild-type (WT) and mutant (KO) samples, each with three replicates. To manually create the design matrix, type:

```
sample.groups <- factor(c("WT", "WT", "WT", "KO", "KO", "KO"),
levels = c("WT", "KO"))
design.mat &lt;- model.matrix(~0 + ~sample.groups)
colnames(design.mat1) ← c("WT", "KO")
```

Similarly, if you want to make a design matrix for three-group comparison (e.g., C, T1, T2 for control, treatment1, treatment2 with two replicates), type:

```
sample.groups <- factor(c("C", "C", "T1", "T1", "T2", "T2"),
levels = c("C", "T1", "T2"))
design.mat &lt;- model.matrix(~0 + sample.groups)
colnames(design.mat2) <- c("C", "T1", "T2")
```

3.4.2 Create Contrast Matrix

For simple experiment designs, design matrix is the only thing needs to be created. However, for those with complex experiment design which could have many ways of comparison, the contrast matrix should also be generated to specify the comparisons need to be performed.

Take the aforementioned three-group experimental design (C, T1, T2 for control, treatment1, treatment2) as example, the contrast matrix which specifies pairwise comparison between each group could be created by typing:

```
contrast.matrix <- makeContrasts(T1-C, T2-C, T2-T1, levels=de-
sign.mat)
```

Similarly, if you are only interested in the differences between the treated groups and control, the contrast matrix could be created by:

```
contrast.matrix <- makeContrasts(T1-C, T2-C, levels=design.
mat)
```

3.4.3 Differential Expression Analysis Using a Linear Model

Once the design matrix (and contrast matrix if necessary) is ready, we can move on to the empirical Bayes analysis which could give more precise estimates of differential genes than traditional approaches like *t*-test. The analysis is carried out by using the command *lmFit()* followed by *eBayes()*. Take the aforementioned three-group experimental design as example, type:

```
fit <- lmFit(eset.filt, contrast.mat)
fit <- eBayes(fit)
```

3.4.4 Report Results

1. Before report the list of differentially expressed genes, it is necessary to map the gene annotation information to "genes" list. To do it, type:

   ```
   fit$genes <- gns [row.names(gns) %in% row.names(fit$t),]
   ```

2. With the *topTable()* function, the differential analysis results could be extracted. By specifying the argument coef, you could determine which comparison results will be reported. Take the three-group experimental design with contrast matrix specifying pair-wise comparison (T1-C, T2-C, T2-T1) as example, you should set coef=1 to get differentially expressed genes between T1 and C groups. Accordingly, coef=2 is for differentially expressed genes between T2 and C groups. To get the top list of differentially expressed genes that pass the specified threshold for log2(fold) (such as 1 as below) by setting "lfc" and p-value (such as BH-adjusted p-value of 0.05 as below) by setting "p.value" between T1 and C groups, type:

   ```
   topTable(fit, coef=1, adjust.method = "BH", sort.by="P",
   lfc = 1, p.value = 0.05, number=10)
   ```

3. To get the list of differential genes, and save them to a local file, type:

```
de.gene = topTable(fit, coef=1, adjust.method = "BH", sort.
by="P", lfc = 1, p.value = 0.05, number=nrow(eset.filt))
write.table(de.gene, file="de_gene.txt", sep="\t", quote=-
FALSE, row.names=FALSE, col.names=TRUE)
```

4. Similarly, to save significantly upregulated and downregulated genes separately, type:

```
up.gene = de.gene[which(de.gene$logFC > 0), ]
down.gene = de.gene[which(de.gene$logFC < 0), ]
write.table(up.gene, file="up_gene.txt", sep="\t", quote=-
FALSE, row.names=FALSE, col.names=TRUE)
write.table(down.gene, file="down_gene.txt", sep="\t", quo-
te=FALSE, row.names=FALSE, col.names=TRUE)
```

3.4.5 Visualize Differentially Expressed Genes

The differentially expressed genes could be plotted in MA plot or Volcano plot, both could be generated using functions provided in limma.

1. To visualize gene expression and highly significantly differentially expressed genes in a MA plot (Fig. 1), and save the figure to a file named "MA_plot.png", type:

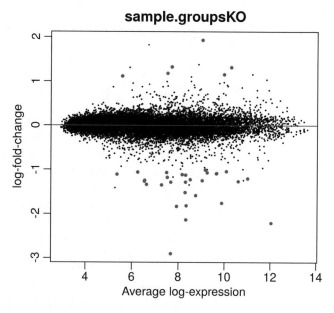

Fig. 1 MA-plot with differentially expressed genes highlighted. The *x*-axis shows the average expression, while *y*-axis shows the log2(fold). The significantly differentially expressed genes are highlighted in red

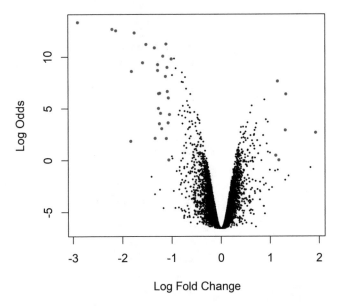

Fig. 2 Volcano plot with differentially expressed genes highlighted. The x-axis shows the log2(fold), while y-axis shows the −log10(p-values). The significantly differentially expressed genes are highlighted in red

```
png(file="MA_plot.png", width=4000, height=3000, res=600)
plotMA(fit,coef=2)
abline(0,0, col="blue")
points(de.gene$AveExpr, de.gene$logFC, col=2, cex=.5,
pch=19)
dev.off()
```

2. Similarly, to visualize differential genes in a Volcano plot using the *volcanoplot()* function (Fig. 2), and save the figure to a file named "volcano_plot.png", type:

```
png(file = "volcano_plot.png", width = 4000, height = 3000,
res = 600)
volcanoplot(fit, coef = 2)
points(de.gene$logFC, de.gene$B, cex=.5, col=2, pch=19)
dev.off()
```

3.5 Downstream Analysis

3.5.1 Clustering and Classification

Gene expression clustering allows an open-ended exploration of the data, without getting lost among the thousands of individual genes [23]. Thus it is one of the standard steps for gene expression analysis.

The R package pheatmap [24] could be used for clustering and heatmap plotting. To be noted, there are multiple ways of distance measurements for clustering, among them Euclidean distance is the most commonly used [25] (*see* **Note 7**).

1. To install and load pheatmap package, type:

```
install.package("pheatmap")
library(pheatmap)
```

2. To get the matrix with expression values for all differential genes, type:

```
de.gene.expr = merge(de.gene, expr[row.names(expr) %in%
row.names(de.gene),], by.x=0, by.y=0, all=TRUE)
```

3. To perform clustering and create a heatmap which shows the expression of differential genes in each sample (Fig. 3), type:

```
png(file = "Fig.de_gene.heatmap.png", width = 3000, height
= 4000, res = 600)
pheatmap(as.matrix(de.gene.expr[,10:17]), scale="row",
labels_row = de.gene.expr$SYMBOL)
dev.off()
```

3.5.2 Gene Ontology Enrichment Analysis

After obtaining the list of differential genes, one analysis is to examine the functional relevance of these genes, by ways like GO enrichment or pathway analysis. The Bioconductor package GOstats [26] could be used for gene set enrichment analysis. To be noted, other resources like DAVID [27] and GSEA [28] are also widely used.

1. To install and load GOstat package, type:

```
biocLite("GOstats")
library(GOstats)
```

2. EntrezIDs are needed by GOstat (*see* **Note 8**). The conversion of probe IDs to Entrez IDs could be carried out easily following steps similar to Subheading 3.1.5. If gene annotation of Entrez IDs has already been performed in previous steps, we could extract Entrez IDs directly by typing:

```
all.ids <- eset.filt$ENTREZID
```

3. To get Entrez IDs of upregulated and downregulated expressed genes, type:

```
up.ids <- up.gene$ENTREZID
down.ids <- down.gene$ENTREZID
```

4. There are three major categories of gene ontology, including "biological process" (BP), "molecular function" (MF), and "cellular component" (CC), each need to be tested separately.

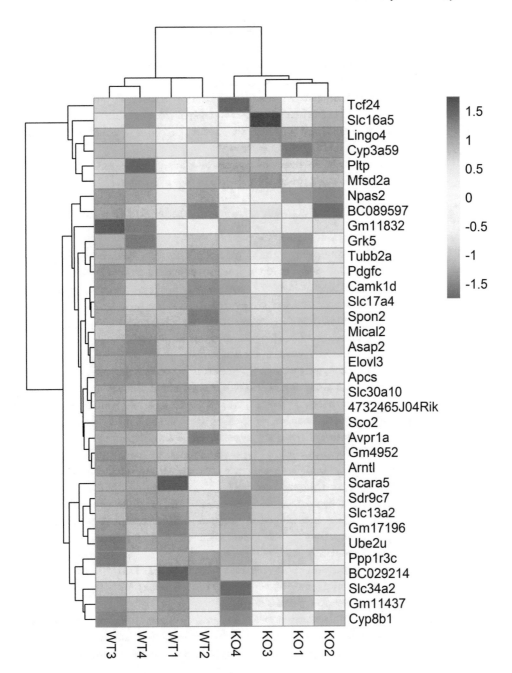

Fig. 3 Heatmap for differentially expressed genes. The expression values are scaled by row. Row z-score is indicated with colors

To get significantly enriched BP terms for upregulated and down-regulated genes respectively, type:

```
up.bp.params <- new(
"GOHyperGParams", geneIds = up.ids, universeGeneIds = all.
ids, annotation = "mogene20sttranscriptcluster.db",
ontology = "BP", pvalueCutoff = 0.05, conditional = FALSE,
```

```
                                          testDirection = "over")
      up.bp.over <- hyperGTest(up.bp.params)
      up.bp.over.df = summary(up.bp.over)
      down.bp.params <- new(
      "GOHyperGParams", geneIds = down.ids, universeGeneIds =
      all.ids, annotation = "mogene20sttranscriptcluster.db",
      ontology = "BP", pvalueCutoff = 0.05, conditional = FALSE,
      testDirection = "over")
      down.bp.over <- hyperGTest(down.bp.params)
      down.bp.over.df = summary(down.bp.over)
```

5. Similarly, to get significantly enriched MF terms, type:

```
      up.mf.params <- new(
      "GOHyperGParams", geneIds = up.ids, universeGeneIds = all.
      ids, annotation = "mogene20sttranscriptcluster.db",
      ontology = "MF", pvalueCutoff = 0.05, conditional = FALSE,
      testDirection = "over")
      up.mf.over <- hyperGTest(up.mf.params)
      up.mf.over.df = summary(up.mf.over)
      down.mf.params <- new(
      "GOHyperGParams", geneIds = down.ids, universeGeneIds =
      all.ids, annotation = "mogene20sttranscriptcluster.db",
      ontology = "MF", pvalueCutoff = 0.05, conditional = FALSE,
      testDirection = "over")
      down.mf.over <- hyperGTest(down.mf.params)
      down.mf.over.df = summary(down.mf.over)
      Similarly, to get significantly enriched CC terms, type:
      up.cc.params <- new(
      "GOHyperGParams", geneIds = up.ids, universeGeneIds = all.
      ids, annotation = "mogene20sttranscriptcluster.db",
      ontology = "CC", pvalueCutoff = 0.05, conditional = FALSE,
      testDirection = "over")
      up.cc.over <- hyperGTest(up.cc.params)
      up.cc.over.df = summary(up.cc.over)
      down.cc.params <- new(
      "GOHyperGParams", geneIds = down.ids, universeGeneIds =
      all.ids, annotation = "mogene20sttranscriptcluster.db",
      ontology = "CC", pvalueCutoff = 0.05, conditional = FALSE,
      testDirection = "over")
      down.cc.over <- hyperGTest(down.cc.params)
      down.cc.over.df = summary(down.cc.over)
```

6. Finally, to save significantly enriched GO terms as local files,
   type:

```
      write.table(up.bp.over.df, file="up_gene.GOstats.enri-
      ched_BP_term.txt",
      row.names = FALSE, sep="\t", quote = FALSE)
      write.table(down.bp.over.df, file="down_gene.GOstats.en-
```

```
riched_BP_term.txt",
row.names = FALSE, sep="\t", quote = FALSE)
write.table(up.bp.over.df,  file="up_gene.GOstats.enri-
ched_BP_term.txt",
row.names = FALSE, sep="\t", quote = FALSE)
write.table(down.bp.over.df,  file="down_gene.GOstats.en-
riched_BP_term.txt",
row.names = FALSE, sep="\t", quote = FALSE)
write.table(up.bp.over.df,  file="up_gene.GOstats.enri-
ched_BP_term.txt",
row.names = FALSE, sep="\t", quote = FALSE)
write.table(down.bp.over.df,  file="down_gene.GOstats.en-
riched_BP_term.txt",
row.names = FALSE, sep="\t", quote = FALSE)
```

4 Notes

1. For researchers prefer to use Affymetrix Power Tools (APT) which is a collection of command line programs for analyzing and working with Affymetrix microarray data, the corresponding annotation files could be downloaded from Affymetrix website freely (http://www.affymetrix.com/support/technical/annotationfilesmain.affx).

2. The CEL file is the raw data file for the Affymetrix microarray. It stores the results of the intensity information for each feature on the microarray, such as the intensity value and the standard deviation of the intensity.

3. The installation of some packages may depend on other packages, which usually will be installed automatically. However, we noticed that some dependent packages, such as "XML" and "openssl" cannot be installed in R successfully. Such problem could usually be solved by install the corresponding package to the computer in advance. For example, in Ubuntu OS, openssl could be installed by the command "apt-get install openssl-dev". After that, openssl could be installed in R successfully.

4. There are a variety of algorithms for microarray data normalization. For their differences, please refer to [11].

5. ExpressionSet is the object defined in the Bioconductor Biobase package for loading and manipulating microarray data in R. It combines several different sources of information, including expression data from microarray experiments, "meta-data" describing samples, annotations about the features on the chip or technology used for the experiment, information related to the protocol used for processing each sample, and a flexible structure to describe the experiment.

6. SAM and RankProduct are specifically designed for the comparison between two groups, while limma provides more flexible choices for experiments with complex design.

7. There are a variety of distance measurements that could be used for clustering. For their differences, please refer to [25].

8. Unique IDs, such as ENTREZID, is good for downstream analysis. Gene symbol is not unique.

Acknowledgments

This work was supported by a Natural Science Funding of Shenzhen (JCYJ201607115221141) and a Shenzhen Peacock Plan fund (827-000116) to YW. The funders had no role in study design, data collection and analysis, decision to publish, or preparation of the manuscript.

References

1. Schena M, Shalon D, Davis RW, Brown PO (1995) Quantitative monitoring of gene expression patterns with a complementary DNA microarray. Science 270(5235):467–470

2. Allison DB, Cui X, Page GP, Sabripour M (2006) Microarray data analysis: from disarray to consolidation and consensus. Nat Rev Genet 7 (1):55–65. https://doi.org/10.1038/nrg1749

3. Hoheisel JD (2006) Microarray technology: beyond transcript profiling and genotype analysis. Nat Rev Genet 7(3):200–210. https://doi.org/10.1038/nrg1809

4. Canales RD, Luo Y, Willey JC, Austermiller B, Barbacioru CC, Boysen C, Hunkapiller K, Jensen RV, Knight CR, Lee KY, Ma Y, Maqsodi B, Papallo A, Peters EH, Poulter K, Ruppel PL, Samaha RR, Shi L, Yang W, Zhang L, Goodsaid FM (2006) Evaluation of DNA microarray results with quantitative gene expression platforms. Nat Biotechnol 24(9):1115–1122. https://doi.org/10.1038/nbt1236

5. Malone JH, Oliver B (2011) Microarrays, deep sequencing and the true measure of the transcriptome. BMC Biol 9:34. https://doi.org/10.1186/1741-7007-9-34

6. Taylor S, Huang Y, Mallett G, Stathopoulou C, Felizardo TC, Sun MA, Martin EL, Zhu N, Woodward EL, Elias MS, Scott J, Reynolds NJ, Paul WE, Fowler DH, Amarnath S (2017) PD-1 regulates KLRG1+ group 2 innate lymphoid cells. J Exp Med 214 (6):1663–1678. https://doi.org/10.1084/jem.20161653

7. The Cancer Genome Atlas Research Network, Weinstein JN, Collisson EA, Mills GB, Shaw KR, Ozenberger BA, Ellrott K, Shmulevich I, Sander C, Stuart JM (2013) The Cancer Genome Atlas Pan-Cancer analysis project. Nat Genet 45(10):1113–1120. https://doi.org/10.1038/ng.2764

8. Kauffmann A, Gentleman R, Huber W (2009) arrayQualityMetrics – a bioconductor package for quality assessment of microarray data. Bioinformatics 25(3):415–416. https://doi.org/10.1093/bioinformatics/btn647

9. Eijssen LM, Jaillard M, Adriaens ME, Gaj S, de Groot PJ, Muller M, Evelo CT (2013) User-friendly solutions for microarray quality control and pre-processing on ArrayAnalysis.org. Nucleic Acids Res 41(Web Server issue): W71–W76. https://doi.org/10.1093/nar/gkt293

10. Wilson CL, Miller CJ (2005) Simpleaffy: a BioConductor package for Affymetrix Quality Control and data analysis. Bioinformatics 21 (18):3683–3685. https://doi.org/10.1093/bioinformatics/bti605

11. Lim WK, Wang K, Lefebvre C, Califano A (2007) Comparative analysis of microarray normalization procedures: effects on reverse engineering gene networks. Bioinformatics 23 (13):i282–i288. https://doi.org/10.1093/bioinformatics/btm201

12. Tusher VG, Tibshirani R, Chu G (2001) Significance analysis of microarrays applied to the ionizing radiation response. Proc Natl Acad Sci

U S A 98(9):5116–5121. https://doi.org/10.1073/pnas.091062498

13. Breitling R, Armengaud P, Amtmann A, Herzyk P (2004) Rank products: a simple, yet powerful, new method to detect differentially regulated genes in replicated microarray experiments. FEBS Lett 573(1-3):83–92. https://doi.org/10.1016/j.febslet.2004.07.055

14. Ritchie ME, Phipson B, Wu D, Hu Y, Law CW, Shi W, Smyth GK (2015) limma powers differential expression analyses for RNA-sequencing and microarray studies. Nucleic Acids Res 43(7):e47. https://doi.org/10.1093/nar/gkv007

15. Huber W, Carey VJ, Gentleman R, Anders S, Carlson M, Carvalho BS, Bravo HC, Davis S, Gatto L, Girke T, Gottardo R, Hahne F, Hansen KD, Irizarry RA, Lawrence M, Love MI, MacDonald J, Obenchain V, Oles AK, Pages H, Reyes A, Shannon P, Smyth GK, Tenenbaum D, Waldron L, Morgan M (2015) Orchestrating high-throughput genomic analysis with Bioconductor. Nat Methods 12(2):115–121. https://doi.org/10.1038/nmeth.3252

16. Carvalho B (2015) pd.mogene.2.0.st: Platform Design Info for Affymetrix MoGene-2_0-st. R package version 3141

17. MacDonald JW (2016) mogene20sttranscriptcluster.db: Affymetrix mogene20 annotation data (chip mogene20sttranscriptcluster). R package version 850

18. Carvalho BS, Irizarry RA (2010) A framework for oligonucleotide microarray preprocessing. Bioinformatics 26(19):2363–2367. https://doi.org/10.1093/bioinformatics/btq431

19. Quackenbush J (2002) Microarray data normalization and transformation. Nat Genet 32(Suppl):496–501. https://doi.org/10.1038/ng1032

20. Bourgon R, Gentleman R, Huber W (2010) Independent filtering increases detection power for high-throughput experiments. Proc Natl Acad Sci U S A 107(21):9546–9551. https://doi.org/10.1073/pnas.0914005107

21. Hackstadt AJ, Hess AM (2009) Filtering for increased power for microarray data analysis. BMC Bioinformatics 10:11. https://doi.org/10.1186/1471-2105-10-11

22. Gentleman R, Carey V, Huber W, Hahne F (2016) genefilter: methods for filtering genes from high-throughput experiments. R package version 1560

23. D'Haeseleer P (2005) How does gene expression clustering work? Nat Biotechnol 23(12):1499–1501. https://doi.org/10.1038/nbt1205-1499

24. Kolde R (2015) pheatmap: Pretty Heatmaps. R package version 108

25. Jaskowiak PA, Campello RJ, Costa IG (2014) On the selection of appropriate distances for gene expression data clustering. BMC Bioinformatics 15(Suppl 2):S2. https://doi.org/10.1186/1471-2105-15-S2-S2

26. Falcon S, Gentleman R (2007) Using GOstats to test gene lists for GO term association. Bioinformatics 23(2):257–258. https://doi.org/10.1093/bioinformatics/btl567

27. Huang d W, Sherman BT, Lempicki RA (2009) Systematic and integrative analysis of large gene lists using DAVID bioinformatics resources. Nat Protoc 4(1):44–57. https://doi.org/10.1038/nprot.2008.211

28. Subramanian A, Tamayo P, Mootha VK, Mukherjee S, Ebert BL, Gillette MA, Paulovich A, Pomeroy SL, Golub TR, Lander ES, Mesirov JP (2005) Gene set enrichment analysis: a knowledge-based approach for interpreting genome-wide expression profiles. Proc Natl Acad Sci U S A 102(43):15545–15550. https://doi.org/10.1073/pnas.0506580102

Check for updates

Chapter 3

Pathway and Network Analysis of Differentially Expressed Genes in Transcriptomes

Qianli Huang, Ming-an Sun, and Ping Yan

Abstract

In recent years, transcriptome sequencing has become very popular, encompassing a wide variety of applications from simple mRNA profiling to discovery and analysis of the entire transcriptome. One of the most common aims of transcriptome sequencing is to identify genes that are differentially expressed (DE) between two or more biological conditions, and to infer associated pathways and gene networks from expression profiles. It can provide avenues for further systematic investigation into potential biologic mechanisms. Gene Set (GS) enrichment analysis is a popular approach to identify pathways or sets of genes that are significantly enriched in the context of differentially expressed genes. However, the approach considers a pathway as a simple gene collection disregarding knowledge of gene or protein interactions. In contrast, topology-based methods integrate the topological structure of a pathway and gene network into the analysis. To provide a panoramic view of such approaches, this chapter demonstrates several recent computational workflows, including gene set enrichment and topology-based methods, for analysis of the DE pathways and gene networks from transcriptome-wide sequencing data.

Key words Transcriptome, RNA-Seq, Microarray, Pathway, Network, Topology, Enrichment analysis

1 Introduction

Transcriptome data are increasing in both volume and variety, which facilitates data mining in system level greatly [1]. A large number of approaches/tools have been developed to detect pathways that are significantly altered between different experimental conditions [2, 3]. These methods can mainly be divided into two categories according to the way by which a pathway is handled in enrichment analysis. The traditional approaches consider pathways as unstructured gene sets and omit known knowledge of the gene and protein interactions. Methods commonly called gene set (GS) analysis are classified as this type. In contrast, in pathway topology-based approaches, the topological structure of a pathway is represented as a graph with nodes (genes or proteins) and edges

Yejun Wang and Ming-an Sun (eds.), *Transcriptome Data Analysis: Methods and Protocols*, Methods in Molecular Biology, vol. 1751, https://doi.org/10.1007/978-1-4939-7710-9_3, © Springer Science+Business Media, LLC 2018

(interactions between genes/proteins), and the pathways' graphical/topological features are integrated into analysis.

Among the methods not using pathway structure, Gene Set Enrichment Analysis (GSEA) proposed by Subramanian et al. is most popular [4]. It determines whether a functionally related set of genes express differentially (enrichment or deletion) under different experimental conditions. As a standard method in the last decade, GSEA has inspired the development of various statistical tests for identifying differentially expressed (DE) gene sets [5]. Several statistical tests are usually employed, such as Fisher's exact, Kolmogorov-Smirnov (KS), Wilcoxon signed rank and Bootstrapping tests. For instance, the DAVID tool (Database for Annotation, Visualization and Integrated Discovery) is based on Fisher's exact test [6]. Although various statistical tests were also implemented in other tools (such as GOStat and SAFE) for significance analysis of functional categories [7, 8], here, we mainly focus on the packages involved in detection of the affected pathways from differentially expressed GS. To demonstrate the GS based analysis approaches, we chose several packages using the statistical programming language R [9], including: GSEA which is based on KS test [10], PATHChange package combining three different tests including Bootstrapping, Fisher's exact and Wilcoxon signed rank tests [11]. For all three statistical tests, the null hypothesis is the same "not differentially expressed pathway" with the alternative hypothesis of "differentially expressed pathway".

For the pathway topology-based (PT-based) methods, SPIA (Signaling Pathway Impact Analysis) proposed by Draghici et al. is one of the earliest tools [12]. Since then, this type of approaches has become popular and several similar methods were developed in recent years [13]. For example, iPathwayGuide is a web-based tool adopting impact analysis to identify the impacted pathways [14]. The PWEA (Pathway Enrichment Analysis) and PRS (Pathway Regulation Score) are standalone applications implemented in programming language C++ and MATLAB, respectively [15, 16]. Packages are also developed with other programming languages, e.g., R, such as TopologyGSA, clipper, DEGraph, SPIA and pathDESeq [12, 17–20]. Simultaneous application of different methods and comparison of the results often appears time-consuming, cumbersome and prone to clerical errors due to the need for repeated data conversion and transfer. Fortunately, the R/Bioconductor package Graphite provides a common interface to four topology-based pathway analysis methods (TopologyGSA, clipper, DEGraph and SPIA), which allows the user to perform these analyses directly over the provided networks [21]. In this chapter, for demonstration of the PT-based methods, we mainly focus on the application of Graphite and pathDESeq packages.

2 Materials

2.1 Installation of R Packages

To perform pathway analysis of gene expression data from microarray and RNA-Seq technologies, all the methods applied in this chapter are implemented in R language. The package could be installed from CRAN (https://cran.r-project.org/), Bioconductor (https://www.bioconductor.org/) or GitHub (https://github.com/). The package "devtools" enables installing packages from GitHub and should be installed in the first place (*see* **Note 1**). Install a package (e.g., "GEOquery") from Github with the following commands:

```
> install.packages("devtools")
> library("devtools")
> install_github('GEOquery','seandavi')
```

2.2 Expression Data

Gene expression datasets curated in Gene Expression Omnibus (GEO) database [22] are downloaded for analysis as specified in context of Methods. GEOquery provided an easy way to access GEO data [23]. Here, an example was shown to download a data matrix (e.g., "GDS3837") from GEO with GEOquery (*see* **Note 2**).

1. Install "GEOquery" and download a GEO dataset:

```
> source("http://bioconductor.org/biocLite.R")
> biocLite("GEOquery")
> library(GEOquery)
> gds <- getGEO( "GDS3837", AnnotGPL = TRUE, destdir=".")
```

2. Get the GPL annotation and inspect the table of GPL annotation object:

```
> gpl <- getGEO(Meta(gds)$platform)
> Meta(gpl)$title
> colnames(Table(gpl))
```

3. Convert a GDS data structure to BioConductor data structure and get expression data:

```
> eset <- GDS2eSet(gds)
> expSet <- exprs(eset)
```

2.3 Pathway/Gene Set Data

There are a large number of metabolic and signaling pathway databases, such as KEGG, PathwayCommons and Reactome [24–26]. Tools such as Graphite and PaxtoolsR have also been developed to download the pathway bundle [21, 27]. Molecular Signatures Database (MSigDB) is one of the most widely used databases of gene sets, which included more than 10,000 gene sets [28]. In the chapter, to reduce the computational complexity of the analysis, only part of pathways is selected. An example using the R package MSigDB to download pathway data is shown below.

1. Install the package MSigDB directly from github:

```
> library(devtools)
> devtools::install_github('oganm/MSigDB')
> library(MSigDB)
```

2. Navigate the pathway information:

```
> names(MSigDB)
> head(names(MSigDB$C2_CURATED))
> getMSigInfo("KEGG_GALACTOSE_METABOLISM")
```

3. Save the pathway information to the local directory:

```
> sink("C2_CURATED.tab")
>  writeLines(unlist(sapply(rbind(names(MSigDB$C2_CURATED),
MSigDB$C2_CURATED), paste, collapse="\t")))
> sink ()
```

3   Methods

3.1   Gene Set Enrichment Based Pathway and Gene Network Analysis

Using pre-defined gene sets that are grouped together according to biological pathways or chromosomal proximity, GSEA evaluates whether gene sets present statistically significant, concordant differences between two biological states [4]. A collection of these priori gene sets can be found in the MSigDB, which are divided into eight major collections, such as curated gene sets from online pathway databases and motif gene sets based on conserved cis-regulatory motifs [29]. GSEA analyzes whether genes in a collection belong to the extreme of the background gene list (a long gene list or genome). If a gene set is at the top (over-expression) or bottom (under-expression), the genes are considered to be associated with biological phenotypic differences. The core of GSEA mainly involves three steps, including calculation of enrichment score (ES), estimation of ES significance, and multi-testing correction.

3.1.1   GSEA

Overview of GSEA

A number of software tools implement the complicated statistical computation required for GSEA, which have been listed in the Broad Institute website: http://software.broadinstitute.org/gsea/downloads.jsp. However, a new R package implementing GSEA with regular updates was introduced here.

Dependencies and Preparations

1. Software installation

The GSEA package can be downloaded from website https://github.com/rskanchi/gsea. To set the file path to your working directory (assuming the working directory is *"D:/Pathway/GSEA"*) and load GSEA in R, open the R console and type:

```
> setwd("D:/Pathway/GSEA")
> source("D:/Pathway/GSEA/gsea.R")
```

2. Input files

   (a) Expression data: The dataset GDS3837 is used as example (https://www.ncbi.nlm.nih.gov/sites/GDSbrowser?acc=GDS3837). The data were generated to mine potential prognostic biomarkers and therapeutic targets for non-smoking female non-small cell lung carcinoma (NSCLC) through collecting 120 paired tumor and adjacent normal lung tissue specimens [30]. A subset of GDS3837 (named "NSCLC.tab") is a data frame with expression data of 20 samples (10 normal vs. 10 tumor). The first column contains gene names while the rest contain gene expression values in samples (*see* **Note 3**).

   (b) Pathway/gene set data: A subset (named "pathways.tab") retrieved from MSigDB is applied. The complete curated gene sets can be downloaded from Broad Institute (http://software.broadinstitute.org/gsea/downloads.jsp). The file "pathways.tab" is tab delimited, with pathway/gene sets represented in rows (*see* **Note 3**).

3. Preprocessing of the gene expression and pathway/gene set data
   It is necessary to read the aforementioned input files into R and convert them to variables as the input arguments for the subsequent functions.

   (a) Preprocessing of the gene expression data
   The function "get.ExpressionData" in gsea.R extracts the gene expression and phenotype labels from the expression data and reorganizes them into a list file with three objects, including a numeric $N \times k$ matrix of expression data, a vector of phenotypic labels, and a vector of gene labels (which is the same as the row names of $N \times k$ matrix output). The function "str()" can be used to compactly display the internal structure of list file.

```
> data <- read.delim("NSCLC.tab", header=FALSE, row.names=1,
stringsAsFactors = FALSE)
> tempData <- get.ExpressionData(data)
> str(tempData)
> exprData <- tempData$exprData;
> phenLabels <- tempData$phenLabels
```

   (b) Preprocessing of the pathway/gene set data
   According to the primary pathway/gene set data, a matrix of pathway/gene should be constructed. In the matrix, the row

names are set as pathway/gene set names, and each row carries names of genes in the corresponding pathway. The column names are laid with the index of specific gene in the line.

```
> nCol <- max (count.fields("pathways.tab", sep = "\t"), na.rm
= TRUE)
> pathways <- read.delim ("pathways.tab", header = FALSE, fill
= TRUE, col.names = 1:nCol)
> rownames(pathways) <- pathways [,1]
> pathways <- pathways [, -(1:2)]
```

Identification of Pathways/ Gene Sets with Significant Expression Difference

Based on the reorganized datasets (*exprData, phenLabels and pathways*), the function "compute.NES" can identify pathways/gene sets with significant expression difference.

```
> myRes <- compute.NES (exprData, phenLabels, pathways, min-
Genes = 15, rankMetric = "t-statistic", p = 1, nperm = 1000, pi
= NULL, computeMinpathways = TRUE)
```

Specifically, the argument *minGenes* designates the minimum number of genes harbored by specific pathway for further analysis, and the *nperm* defines the number of permutations to build the null distributions for assessing the statistical significance of the enrichment score (default 1000). These parameters can be adjusted to meet specific requirements (*see* **Note 4**).

After this step, the results (myRes, an object of list) will be generated and saved as two files ("pathwayScored.tab" and "geneRanked.tab") in the working directory. The file "pathwayScored. tab" is a dataframe describing the statistical outputs (such as enrichment score (ES), normalized enrichment score (NES), Perm-pval, FWER p value, and FDR q value) of each pathway/gene set. The file "geneRanked.tab" contains the genes and corresponding values in decreasing order measuring the association of each gene with the phenotype.

```
> str(myRes)
> write.table(myRes$NES,quote = FALSE,sep="\t", "pathwayS-
cored.tab")
> write.table(myRes$rankedL,quote = FALSE,sep="\t", "geneR-
anked.tab")
```

3.1.2 PATHChange

Overview of PATHChange

PATHChange is an R package that detects differentially expressed pathways in transcriptomic data [9, 11]. To facilitate the evaluation of significant alterations of pathways and to reduce possible false discoveries, PATHChange combines three different statistical tests, including Bootstrapping, Fisher's exact and Wilcoxon signed rank tests [11]. The standard analysis process of the PATHChange includes four steps: (a) expression data preprocessing and expression variation evaluation [31]; (b) pathway data preprocessing; (c) pathway activity analysis; (d) comparison of the results from these three methods with Venn diagrams, and this final step is optional. For the example illustrated in this section, each file produced by PATHChange package is saved in the temporary folder.

Dependencies and Preparations

1. Software installation
The package can be installed and loaded as followed.

```
> install.packages("PATHChange")
> library("PATHChange")
```

2. Input files
Here, the gene data file (named "genes.txt"), the pathway data file (named "pathways.txt") and the expression data file (named "eDat.csv") are all retrieved from example data in the package PATHChange (https://github.com/cran/PATHChange). Their formats are briefly described as follows.

(a) Pathway data: This is a text formatted file with two columns: 'Pathway' and 'ApprovedSymbol'. Each row of the file starts with the pathway/gene set name followed by a space, and then a gene name in that pathway/gene set. There are a large number of databases curating metabolic and signaling pathways, such as KEGG, PathwayCommons and Reactome [24–26], which may be considered for checking alterations.

(b) Gene data: This is a text formatted file organized in a single column named "ApprovedSymbol", which contains all gene members in all tested pathways.

(c) Expression data: This file comprises of an expression matrix and has been saved as a comma-separated values format (*. csv; the function in the PATHChange uses "/" *as* mark of separation). The first row of this file contains the labels for each column, including probes, genes and the expression level of the gene in different conditions/samples. In other words, the gene expression matrix (N probes/genes $\times$ k conditions/samples) is available from the second row onwards with the probe and gene name in the first and second column followed by k expression values for the conditions/samples (*see* **Note 5**).

Preprocessing Expression Data with PATHChangeDat Function

Firstly, PATHChangeDat detects the experimental conditions provided in expression files which can be retrieved from GEO, and confirms the sample/control combinations for further comparative analyses based on users' choice. Then, it calculates the mean expression value of each gene in sample combinations. Because the repeated genes may affect the probability of choosing each gene in Bootstrap algorithm, the average expression level will also be used as a substitute for these genes. Here, we use the dataset GSE35972 from GEO as example.

```
> PATHChangeDat(eDat = eDat, DataSet = "GSE35972", NumbSample
= 6, Genes = Genes, HistComp = FALSE, hc = c("untreated",
"treated with"), writeRDS = FALSE)
```

For the parameters/arguments, *NumbSample* represents the number of samples in dataset. If the users already know which sample types are used for comparison, they can select *Hist-Comp=FALSE* and set the sample types in the argument *hc*. For instance, *hc=c("untreated", "treated with")* indicates that comparison will be performed between "untreated" and "treated with" sample combinations. The result of PATHChangeDat is a list file (named "MeanData.rds") demonstrating the mean expression value of each gene.

```
> require(rlist)
> MeanData <- list.load(file.path(tempdir(), "MeanData.rds"))
> write.table (MeanData, quote = FALSE, sep = "\t", "D:/
Pathway/PATHChange/MeanData.tab")
```

Preprocessing Pathways with PATHChangeList Function

Based on the pathway data provided, this function organizes the different pathways and carried genes separately to a list file (named "path.rds").

```
> PATHChangeList(filePathway = filePathway, writeRDS = FALSE)
> path <- list.load(file.path(tempdir(), "path.rds"))
> head(path)
```

Detection of Differentially Expressed Pathways with PATHChange Function

Based on the primary data processed in foregoing steps, this function detects differentially expressed pathways with Bootstrapping, Fisher's exact and Wilcoxon signed-rank tests. The results are displayed in a file (.csv) with five columns, including "Pathway" representing the considered pathway name, "Activity" denoting the calculated pathway activity and the p-values resulting from three statistical tests. The altered pathways can be used for further comparative analyses and visualization.

```
> PATHChange(path = path, MeanData = MeanData, writeCSV =
TRUE, writeRDS = FALSE, destDIR = " D:/Pathway/PATHChange/")
```

Specifically, the parameter/argument *path* is the list of pathways previously generated by the function PATHChangeList. The *MeanData* indicates the mean expression value of each gene calculated with the function PATHChangeDat.

3.2 Topology Based Pathway and Gene Network Analysis

3.2.1 pathDESeq

Overview of pathDESeq

pathDESeq is a pathway-based approach of DE analysis for RNA-Seq gene expression data [17]. To improve sensitivity and specificity for detecting differentially expressed genes, pathDESeq integrates known biological pathways and interaction information to the Markov Random Field (MRF) method. Compared to other popular R packages for RNA-Seq data analysis, e.g., DESeq, EBSeq, edgeR, NOISeq, etc [32–35], pathDESeq adopts network information and increases the sensitivity. The package can be retrieved from GitHub (https://github.com/MalathiSIDona/pathDESeq).

Dependencies and Preparations

1. Software installation

```
> library("devtools")
> install_github("MalathiSIDona/pathDESeq", build_vignettes=-
TRUE)
> library("pathDESeq")
```

2. Input files

(a) RNA-Seq data: Normalized count data (FPKM/RPKM format [17]) is required as pathDESeq input. A subset of data ("CRC.tab") derived from GSE50760 dataset is used as example [36]. The file "CRC.tab" is a data frame with normalized (FPKM) expression data of 18 samples (9 normal colons vs. 9 primary colorectal cancers). The first column contains gene names while the rest contain gene expression values for each sample.

(b) Reactome pathway data: The gene information in human reactome pathways is retrieved from Reactome pathway database [26]. The unique gene names are deposited in the file named "pathway.tab". Note that only the genes that can be mapped to at least one pathway in the Reactome pathway database are used for further analysis [17]. If needed, other databases that contain biological pathway information can also be combined to filter the genes.

(c) Gene-gene interaction data: The curated gene-gene interactions for human are downloaded from BioGRID database [37] and saved in the file "Biogrid.tab". It is a data frame with each row representing a gene-gene interaction pair and two columns carrying the Gene.1 and Gene.2 of the interaction pair respectively. In the analysis, the gene-gene interaction data are applied to form the neighborhood structure. If needed, other databases that harbor gene network/interaction information can also be combined.

Data Preprocessing

Only the genes mapped to at least one pathway are used for further pathway analysis in the package pathDESeq. Moreover, the expression data file may contain duplicate gene names, and the expression values could be missing for some genes. So, the data should be preprocessed.

First, read the required data to R environment:

```
> Exp_dataset <- read.table("CRC.tab", header = TRUE, string-
sAsFactors = FALSE, sep='\t')
> Path_Rectome <- read.table("pathway.tab", stringsAsFactors
= FALSE, sep = '\t')
> biogrid <- read.table("Biogrid.tab", header = TRUE, string-
sAsFactors = FALSE, sep = '\t')
```

Keep the genes (in expression data) that are recalled from Reactome pathway data:

```
> Exp_dataset1 <- data.frame (subset(Exp_dataset, Exp_dataset
$genes %in% Path_Rectome$V1))
```

Remove rows with duplicate gene names:

```
> Exp_dataset2 <- Exp_dataset1[!duplicated(Exp_dataset1
$genes), ]
```

It is needed to remove the rows (genes) with missing or zero expression values:

```
> Exp_dataset3 <- Exp_dataset2[rowSums(is.na(Exp_dataset2))
== 0,]
> Exp_dataset4 <- Exp_dataset3[rowSums(Exp_dataset3[,-1]) >
0,]
```

Estimation of Differential Expressed Genes with PGBMRF Model

This function is a wrapper function, which consists of *ttest, neib-Mat, pgbEst* and *estDE* sub-functions with Iterative Conditional Mode (ICM) algorithm to perform the PGBMRF analysis. The function performs two independent sample *t* tests to obtain initial DE states for given genes and create the neighborhood matrix based on available gene interaction information, followed by estimation of the parameters for PGBMRF model and the DE states for given genes using ICM algorithm with three iterative steps until the estimated DE states converge.

```
> pgbmrfICM(data = Exp_dataset4, interactions = biogrid, m =
9, n = 9, sig = 0.05, k = 40, pgb.start = c(log(10), log(0.2),
log(2), log(3)), iterations = 12)
```

For the arguments, *data* and *interactions* originate from above input files. *m* and *n* specify the number of replicates for the control and treatment group, respectively. *sig, k, pgb.start* and *iterations* denote the level of significance, the number of Gaussian quadrature points, a vector of initial parameters for the Poisson-Gamma-Beta model and the maximum number of ICM iterations, respectively. Note that all the parameters are assigned with default values and they can be altered according to users' preference. Afterwards, the following result files will be generated as expected in the working directory (*see* **Note 6**).

Detection of Enriched Pathways for Differentially Expressed Genes

With MRF method that utilizes prior knowledge of biological pathways and interaction, differentially expressed (DE) genes can be identified with improved sensitivity and specificity from RNA-Seq data. Subsequently, DAVID or other tools can be used to find the enriched pathways [6, 17]. Here, an alternative method named FunEnrich (https://github.com/galanisl/FunEnrich) is adopted to execute the pathway enrichment analyses.

```
> library("devtools")
> source("https://bioconductor.org/biocLite.R")
> biocLite("reactome.db")
> install_github("galanisl/FunEnrich")
> library("FunEnrich")
```

The FunEnrich requires two gene lists (gene list of "interest" and "background") as inputs. Here, the up- (UR) and down-regulated (DR) genes identified with PGBMRF are combined as the gene list of interest. All genes in Human Reactome pathways are used as background:

```
> DR_gene <- read.table("PGBMRF identified DR genes.txt",
header = FALSE, stringsAsFactors = FALSE, sep = '\t')
> UR_gene <- read.table("PGBMRF identified UR genes.txt",
header = FALSE, stringsAsFactors = FALSE, sep = '\t')
> DE_total <- rbind(DR_gene, UR_gene)
> Path_Rectome <- read.table("pathway.tab", stringsAsFactors
= FALSE, sep = '\t')
```

Subsequently, enrichment analysis is conducted with the function *fun_enrich*. Note that the *gene.list* should be a perfect subset of the *background* and *id.type* should be one of *ENTREZID* (default), *SYMBOL* (GENE SYMBOLs) and *UNIPROT* accessions.

```
> enriched <- fun_enrich(gene.list = DE_total[-1,], back-
ground = Path_Rectome[-1,], id.type = "SYMBOL", benjamini =
FALSE)
> str(enriched)
> write.table(enriched$bp, quote = FALSE, sep = "\t", "en-
riched_bp.tab")
```

```
> write.table(enriched$cc, quote = FALSE, sep = "\t", "en-
riched_cc.tab")
> write.table(enriched$mf, quote = FALSE, sep = "\t", "en-
riched_mf.tab")
> write.table(enriched$reactome, quote = FALSE, sep = "\t",
"enriched_reactome.tab")
> plot_fun_enrich(enr = enriched, aspect = "ALL", benjamini
= F, top = 5, char_per_line = 80)
```

The result (*enriched*, an object of list) will be generated. It can be divided into four files (named "enriched_bp.tab", "enriched_cc.tab", "enriched_mf.tab" and "enriched_reactome.tab"), representing enriched biological process, cellular component, molecular functions and REACTOME pathways, respectively. The function *plot_fun_enrich* generates a bar plot that focuses on the top enriched terms (such as *top* = 5) of one or all categories.

3.2.2 Graphite

Overview of Graphite

Graphite (GRAPH Interaction from pathway Topological Environment) is an R package performing topology-based gene set analyses through conversion of pathway topology to a gene/protein network [21, 38]. It reconstructs the gene-gene networks by integrating six pathway databases and taking into account the protein complexes, gene families and compound-mediated interactions. Interactions are included not only involving genes or their product but also other chemical compounds (e.g., calcium ions). The package provides options to: (1) construct networks based on six databases, including KEGG, Biocarta (http://www.biocarta.com), Reactome, NCI/Nature Pathway Interaction Database, HumanCyc, and Panther [25, 26, 39–41]; (2) discriminate among different types of gene groups from 14 species since the version 1.14; (3) propagate pathway signal through the compound-mediated interactions; (4) allow the selection of edge attributes and the mapping of node identifiers to EntrezGene IDs and HUGO Symbols [42, 43]; (4) the last but most important point, run SPIA, DEGraph, CliPPER and topologyGSA analyses directly on networks constructed by Graphite [12, 19, 20, 38]. The Graphite package is available in Bioconductor: http://bioconductor.org/packages/devel/bioc/html/graphite.html.

Dependencies and Preparations

1. Software installation

Install and load the latest version of the package by entering in R console:

```
> source("https://bioconductor.org/biocLite.R")
> biocLite("graphite")
> library(graph)
> library(graphite)
```

Four packages (*SPIA*, *DEGraph*, *topologyGSA* and *clipper*), which are involved in identification of the most affected pathways under the study based on pathways topology analysis, should also be installed:

```
> biocLite(c("SPIA", "DEGraph", "topologyGSA", "clipper"))
```

2. Input files
    (a) Pathway data:
        The package can integrate the pathways from six public databases (KEGG, Reactome, BioCarta, NCI, Panther and HumanCyc) and convert them to gene network. The data can be called using function *pathways()*. The names of interested species and the pathway database are required (KEGG as an example):

```
> humanKEGG <- pathways("hsapiens", "kegg")
> names(humanKEGG)[1:10]
> p <- humanKEGG[["Adherens junction"]]
> p
```

All the six databases are available for human in the package. For other organisms, the pathway data are not always distributed. The list of available pathway databases can be retrieved through "pathwayDatabases()", which returns a data frame with two columns: *species* and *database.*

```
> pathwayDatabases()
```

    (b) Expression data:
        Because four types of methods (SPIA, DEGraph, topologyGSA and clipper) are integrated in Graphite package, different types of input files are needed. For instance, expression profiles are used for the multivariable methods, such as topologyGSA. Some other methods use the gene-level statistics like log fold-change. The specific requirements for file formats are described in corresponding sections.

Different Topology-Based Pathway Analysis Approaches

1. SPIA

The SPIA is one of the most well-known topology-based pathway analysis methods [12]. It evaluates two probabilities. The first probability (differentially expressed genes belonging to a pathway) is calculated through a regular overrepresentation analysis, and the second one assumes that the genes located in different positions of a pathway have different perturbation factors. Then, global *p*-value, which is used to rank the pathways, is obtained by combining the two probabilities. Three arguments are needed as its inputs: a named vector (with Entrez Gene IDs) containing log2 fold-changes of the differentially expressed genes, a vector with the Entrez IDs in the reference set (for a microarray experiment, the set will contain all genes present on the specific array used for the experiment), and a list of pathways as mentioned. For instance:

Load the package and example dataset:

```
> library(SPIA)
> data(colorectalcancer)
```

Install and load Affymetrix Human Genome U133 Plus 2.0 Array annotation data (chip hgu133plus2):

```
> biocLite("hgu133plus2.db")
> library(hgu133plus2.db)
```

Using the example data, obtain the named vector containing log2 fold-changes of the differentially expressed genes and a vector with the Entrez IDs matched to the expression dataset:

```
> x <- hgu133plus2ENTREZID
> top$ENTREZ <- unlist(as.list(x[top$ID]))
> top <- top[!is.na(top$ENTREZ), ]
> top <- top[!duplicated(top$ENTREZ), ]
> tg1 <- top[top$adj.P.Val < 0.05, ]
> DE_Colorectal = tg1$logFC
> names(DE_Colorectal) <- as.vector(tg1$ENTREZ)
> ALL_Colorectal <- top$ENTREZ
```

Using the database Reactome as an example, get a list of pathways. Note that the function prepareSPIA converts the networks to the SPIA-recognized format and should be executed before running SPIA.

```
> b <- pathways("hsapiens", "Reactome")
> prepareSPIA(b[1:20], "path_rect")
```

Run a topology-based analysis on an expression dataset using SPIA:

```
> res_SPIA <- runSPIA(de=DE_Colorectal, all=ALL_Colorectal,
"path_rect")
> write.table(res_SPIA,quote = FALSE,sep="\t", "result_SPIA.
tab")
```

The ranked pathways and various statistical results are deposited in the result file ("result_SPIA.tab"). In particular, pSize is the number of genes in the pathway; NDE is the number of DE genes per pathway; tA is the observed total alteration accumulation in the pathway; pNDE is the probability to observe at least NDE genes on the pathway using a hypergeometric model; pPERT is the probability to observe a total accumulation more extreme than tA only by chance; pG is the *p*-value obtained by combining pNDE and pPERT; pGFdr and pGFWER are the False Discovery Rate and Bonferroni adjusted global *p*-values, respectively. The Status provides how the pathway is perturbed (activated or inhibited).

2. TopologyGSA

TopologyGSA represents a multivariable method in which the expression of genes is modeled with Gausian Graphical Models with covariance matrix reflecting the pathway topology [20]. It uses the Iterative Proportional Scaling algorithm to estimate the covariance matrices. The testing procedure is a two-step process. First, the equality of covariance matrices is tested via a likelihood ratio test. When the null hypothesis of equality of covariance matrices is not rejected, the differential expression is tested via multivariate analysis of variance. When the covariance matrices are not equal, Behrens-Fisher method is employed, which tests the equality of means in a two-sample problem with unequal covariance matrices. Five arguments are needed as its inputs, including: *PathwayList*, which specifies a list of Pathways or a single Pathway object; *test*, which determines the type of test used by topologyGSA; *exp1*, which contains the Experiment matrix (of the first group) with each gene in one column; *exp2*, which contains the Experiment matrix (of the second group) with each gene in one column; *alpha*, which represents the significance level of the test. For instance,

```
> library(topologyGSA)
> data(examples)
> k <- pathways("hsapiens", "kegg")
> p <- convertIdentifiers(k[["Fc epsilon RI signaling path-
way"]], "symbol")
```

The pathway list can be a list of pathways or a single pathway. *"symbol"* is a string describing the type of the identifier. The values can be "entrez", "symbol" or one of the columns provided by an annotation package (for example, "UNIPROT").

```
> runTopologyGSA(p, "var", y1, y2, 0.05)
```

The results are demonstrated in a list with the pathway analyses and the list of generated errors. Note that the process returns a warning or NULL when the number of genes in common is less than 3 between the expression matrices and the pathway.

3. DEGraph

This method directly assesses whether a particular gene network is differentially expressed between two conditions by assuming the same direction in the differential expression of genes belonging to a pathway [18]. Three arguments are needed as its inputs: *PathwayList*, specifies a list of pathways or a single pathway object, *expr* is an expression matrix with genes in rows and *N* samples in columns, and *Classes* is a vector (length: *N*) indicating the group assignment of the *N* samples.

```
> library(DEGraph)
> data("Loi2008_DEGraphVignette")
> b <- pathways("hsapiens", "biocarta")
> p <- convertIdentifiers(b[["actions of nitric oxide in the
heart"]], "entrez")
> runDEGraph(p, exprLoi2008, classLoi2008 )
```

4. Clipper

This method is similar to the topologyGSA as it uses the same two-step approach. However, the Iterative Proportional Scaling algorithm was substituted with a shrinkage James-Stein-type procedure allowing proper estimates when the number of samples is smaller than that of genes in a pathway [19]. Then, it "clips" the whole pathway for identifying the most affected path in the graph. Four arguments are needed as its inputs: *PathwayList*, *expr* and *Classes* are same as for DEGraph; *method* shows the kind of test to be performed on the cliques and could be either "mean" or "variance". Below, an example is given to explain how to apply the package (with "ALL" dataset from Bioconductor).

```
> source("https://bioconductor.org/biocLite.R")
> biocLite("a4Preproc")
> library(a4Preproc)
> biocLite("hgu95av2.db")
> library(hgu95av2.db)
> library(ALL)
> library(clipper)
> data(ALL)
```

Prepare the required the pathway list from KEGG:

```
> k <- as.list(pathways("hsapiens", "kegg"))
> selected <- k[c("Bladder cancer", "Cytosolic DNA-sensing
pathway")]
```

Preprocess data from the *ALL* and prepare the required expression and group/class files:

```
> pheno <- as(phenoData(ALL), "data.frame")
> samples <- unlist(lapply(c("NEG", "BCR/ABL"), function
(t) {which(grepl("^B\\d*", pheno$BT) & (pheno$mol.biol == t))
[1:10] }))
> classes <- c(rep(1,10), rep(2,10))
> expr <- exprs(ALL)[,samples]
> rownames(expr) <- featureData(addGeneInfo(ALL))$ENTREZID
```

Run a topology based analysis on an expression dataset using *runClipper*:

```
> clipped <- runClipper(selected, expr, classes, "mean",
pathThr = 0.1)
> str(clipped$results)
```

The result provides a list with the results of the pathway analyses and generated errors.

4   Notes

1. When you install R packages, please note that there is difference between "install.packages()" and "install_github()" in the required argument. The "install.packages()" takes package names, while "install_github()" needs not only package names but also repository names. It means that when a package on GitHub is to be installed, its repository name should be provided correctly. As shown in the example, "GEOquery" is a well-known package on GitHub and the repository name is "seandavi". If you think it is trouble to use the repository name of package on GitHub, the package "githubinstall" provides an alternative solution to install packages on GitHub just like "install.packages()" use the following code:

   ```
   > install.packages("githubinstall")
   > library(githubinstall)
   > githubinstall("GEOquery")
   ```

2. When using the function "getGEO()" to download GEO data, please note that the default destination directory for any downloads is "tempdir()". It means that the retrieved file (e.g., "GDS3837.soft.gz") is stored at "tempdir()". You can type "tempdir()" in R Console to get the path of directory. If you would like to save the file for later use, it is necessary to specify a

different directory. Since some GEO files are big, it is a good idea to set a directory especially when your internet connection is slow. Moreover, the GEO data can be converted to BioConductor ExpressionSets and limma MALists (https://github.com/seandavi/GEOquery).

3. For the expression data, the gene expression matrix comprises of expression values of N genes in k samples (N genes × k samples). The first row of the data file contains the experimental labels of the two phenotypic states for k samples. The expression data of N genes are available from the second row onwards with the gene name in the first column followed by k expression values in the column of corresponding samples. Notably, if the gene expression data are retrieved from GEO, the expression data for all the probes should match with a gene symbol/ENTREZ ID or other annotated information. For the pathway data file, each row contains three tab-separated cells of the pathway/gene set name, description of the pathway/gene set, and all the gene names in that pathway/gene set. Note that if you would like to get the pathways from Molecular Signatures Database, registration is required.

4. The default permutation times are set as 1000. It is quite time-consuming so that it is advised to evaluate whether the analysis will complete successfully. It is better to start with a small permutation number such as 10. Once the workflow is running smoothly, the number of permutations can be set according to necessity. Bear in mind that a very large number of permutations are computationally expensive and often infeasible; sometimes, more accurate p-values can be obtained with fewer permutations [44].

5. These input files need to be read into R and converted to a more general form to be passed on as input arguments to different functions in this package. Here, the corresponding commands to read files have been implanted into the functions involved in the package PATHChange, for instance:

```
> GenesSet <- read.table(Genes, header=TRUE)
> Pathway <- read.table(filePathway, header=TRUE)
> eDat <- read.table(eDat, header = TRUE, sep = "/")
```

So, we need to assign the information of input files to corresponding variables as following (assuming that the file path is "*D:/Pathway/PATHChange*").

```
> Genes <- "D:/Pathway/PATHChange/genes.txt"
> filePathway <- "D:/Pathway/PATHChange/Pathways.txt"
> eDat <- "D:/Pathway/PATHChange/eDat.csv"
```

6. The pgbmrfICM function produces six result files. The files are described briefly as below.

   (a) "selected dataset.txt": the gene expression dataset used for the PGBMRF analysis;

   (b) "neib_matrix.txt": the neighbourhood matrix which demonstrates the gene-gene interactions;

   (c) "PGBMRF identified UR genes.txt": up-regulated genes identified by PGBMRF model;

   (d) "PGBMRF identified DR genes.txt": down-regulated genes identified by PGBMRF model;

   (e) "PGBMRF states.txt": the final estimated DE states. For convenience, the three expression states are labeled numerically as 0, 1 and −1 for equally expressed EE, UR and DR genes, respectively.

   (f) "PGBMRF results.txt": a summary table for the PGBMRF analysis.

Acknowledgments

This work was supported by the Fundamental Research Funds for the Central Universities (Grant No. JZ2017YYPY0899). The authors are grateful to the editors and the anonymous reviewers for their valuable suggestions and comments facilitating the improvement of this chapter.

References

1. Conesa A, Madrigal P, Tarazona S, Gomez-Cabrero D, Cervera A, McPherson A, Szcześniak MW, Gaffney DJ, Elo LL, Zhang X, Mortazavi A (2016) A survey of best practices for RNA-Seq data analysis. Genome Biol 17:13. https://doi.org/10.1186/s13059-016-0881-8

2. Bayerlova M, Jung K, Kramer F, Klemm F, Bleckmann A, Beissbarth T (2015) Comparative study on gene set and pathway topology-based enrichment methods. BMC Bioinformatics 16:334. https://doi.org/10.1186/s12859-015-0751-5

3. Jaakkola MK, Elo LL (2016) Empirical comparison of structure-based pathway methods. Brief Bioinform 17(2):336–345. https://doi.org/10.1093/bib/bbv049

4. Subramanian A, Tamayo P, Mootha VK, Mukherjee S, Ebert BL, Gillette MA, Paulovich A, Pomeroy SL, Golub TR, Lander ES, Mesirov JP (2005) Gene set enrichment analysis: a knowledge-based approach for interpreting genome-wide expression profiles. Proc Natl Acad Sci 102(43):15545–15550. https://doi.org/10.1073/pnas.0506580102

5. Nam D, Kim S-Y (2008) Gene-set approach for expression pattern analysis. Brief Bioinform 9(3):189–197

6. Huang d W, Sherman BT, Lempicki RA (2009) Systematic and integrative analysis of large gene lists using DAVID bioinformatics resources. Nat Protoc 4(1):44–57. https://doi.org/10.1038/nprot.2008.211

7. Barry WT, Nobel AB, Wright FA (2005) Significance analysis of functional categories in gene expression studies: a structured permutation approach. Bioinformatics 21(9):1943–1949. https://doi.org/10.1093/bioinformatics/bti260

8. Beissbarth T, Speed TP (2004) GOstat: find statistically overrepresented gene ontologies within a group of genes. Bioinformatics 20(9):1464–1465. https://doi.org/10.1093/bioinformatics/bth088

9. Team RC (2014) R: A language and environment for statistical computing. Vienna, Austria: R Foundation for Statistical Computing 14 (3):279-293.

10. Charmpi K, Ycart B (2015) Weighted Kolmogorov Smirnov testing: an alternative for gene set enrichment analysis. Stat Appl Genet Mol Biol 14. https://doi.org/10.1515/sagmb-2014-0077

11. Fontoura CARS, Castellani G, Mombach JCM (2016) The R implementation of the CRAN package PATHChange, a tool to study genetic pathway alterations in transcriptomic data. Comput Biol Med 78:76–80. https://doi.org/10.1016/j.compbiomed.2016.09.010

12. Draghici S, Khatri P, Tarca AL, Amin K, Done A, Voichita C, Georgescu C, Romero R (2007) A systems biology approach for pathway level analysis. Genome Res 17 (10):1537–1545. https://doi.org/10.1101/gr.6202607

13. Mitrea C, Taghavi Z, Bokanizad B, Hanoudi S, Tagett R, Donato M, Voichiţa C, Drǎghici S (2013) Methods and approaches in the topology-based analysis of biological pathways. Front Physiol 4:278. https://doi.org/10.3389/fphys.2013.00278

14. Ahsan S, Draghici S (2017) Identifying significantly impacted pathways and putative mechanisms with iPathwayGuide. Curr Protoc Bioinformatics 57:7.15.11–17.15.30. https://doi.org/10.1002/cpbi.24

15. Ibrahim M, Jassim S, Cawthorne MA, Langlands K (2014) A MATLAB tool for pathway enrichment using a topology-based pathway regulation score. BMC Bioinformatics 15:358. https://doi.org/10.1186/s12859-014-0358-2

16. Wadi L, Meyer M, Weiser J, Stein LD, Reimand J (2016) Impact of outdated gene annotations on pathway enrichment analysis. Nat Methods 13(9):705–706. https://doi.org/10.1038/nmeth.3963

17. Dona MSI, Prendergast LA, Mathivanan S, Keerthikumar S, Salim A (2017) Powerful differential expression analysis incorporating network topology for next-generation sequencing data. Bioinformatics 33(10):1505–1513. https://doi.org/10.1093/bioinformatics/btw833

18. Jacob L, Neuvial P, Dudoit S (2010) Gains in power from structured two-sample tests of means on graphs. arXiv preprint arXiv:10095173

19. Martini P, Sales G, Massa MS, Chiogna M, Romualdi C (2013) Along signal paths: an empirical gene set approach exploiting pathway topology. Nucleic Acids Res 41(1):e19–e19. https://doi.org/10.1093/nar/gks866

20. Massa MS, Chiogna M, Romualdi C (2010) Gene set analysis exploiting the topology of a pathway. BMC Syst Biol 4:121. https://doi.org/10.1186/1752-0509-4-121

21. Sales G, Calura E, Cavalieri D, Romualdi C (2012) graphite - a Bioconductor package to convert pathway topology to gene network. BMC Bioinformatics 13:20–20. https://doi.org/10.1186/1471-2105-13-20

22. Clough E, Barrett T (2016) The Gene Expression Omnibus database. Methods Mol Biol 1418:93–110. https://doi.org/10.1007/978-1-4939-3578-9_5

23. Davis S, Meltzer PS (2007) GEOquery: a bridge between the Gene Expression Omnibus (GEO) and BioConductor. Bioinformatics 23:1846–1847.

24. Cerami EG, Gross BE, Demir E, Rodchenkov I, Babur O, Anwar N, Schultz N, Bader GD, Sander C (2011) Pathway Commons, a web resource for biological pathway data. Nucleic Acids Res 39(Database): D685–D690. https://doi.org/10.1093/nar/gkq1039

25. Kanehisa M, Furumichi M, Tanabe M, Sato Y, Morishima K (2017) KEGG: new perspectives on genomes, pathways, diseases and drugs. Nucleic Acids Res 45(D1):D353–D361. https://doi.org/10.1093/nar/gkw1092

26. Sidiropoulos K, Viteri G, Sevilla C, Jupe S, Webber M, Orlic-Milacic M, Jassal B, May B, Shamovsky V, Duenas C (2017) Reactome enhanced pathway visualization. Bioinformatics 33(21):3461–3467

27. Luna A, Babur O, Aksoy BA, Demir E, Sander C (2016) PaxtoolsR: pathway analysis in R using Pathway Commons. Bioinformatics 32 (8):1262–1264. https://doi.org/10.1093/bioinformatics/btv733

28. Liberzon A, Birger C, Thorvaldsdóttir H, Ghandi M, Mesirov JP, Tamayo P (2015) The Molecular Signatures Database (MSigDB) hallmark gene set collection. Cell Syst 1 (6):417–425. https://doi.org/10.1016/j.cels.2015.12.004

29. Liberzon A, Subramanian A, Pinchback R, Thorvaldsdóttir H, Tamayo P, Mesirov JP (2011) Molecular signatures database (MSigDB) 3.0. Bioinformatics 27 (12):1739–1740. https://doi.org/10.1093/bioinformatics/btr260

30. Lu TP, Tsai MH, Lee JM, Hsu CP, Chen PC, Lin CW, Shih JY, Yang PC, Hsiao CK, Lai LC, Chuang EY (2010) Identification of a novel biomarker, SEMA5A, for non-small cell lung

carcinoma in nonsmoking women. Cancer Epidemiol Biomarkers Prevent 19 (10):2590–2597. https://doi.org/10.1158/1055-9965.epi-10-0332

31. Barrett T, Wilhite SE, Ledoux P, Evangelista C, Kim IF, Tomashevsky M, Marshall KA, Phillippy KH, Sherman PM, Holko M (2012) NCBI GEO: archive for functional genomics data sets—update. Nucleic Acids Res 41(D1): D991–D995

32. Anders S, Huber W (2010) Differential expression analysis for sequence count data. Genome Biol 11(10):R106. https://doi.org/10.1186/gb-2010-11-10-r106

33. Leng N, Dawson JA, Thomson JA, Ruotti V, Rissman AI, Smits BMG, Haag JD, Gould MN, Stewart RM, Kendziorski C (2013) EBSeq: an empirical Bayes hierarchical model for inference in RNA-Seq experiments. Bioinformatics 29(8):1035–1043. https://doi.org/10.1093/bioinformatics/btt087

34. Robinson MD, McCarthy DJ, Smyth GK (2010) edgeR: a Bioconductor package for differential expression analysis of digital gene expression data. Bioinformatics 26 (1):139–140. https://doi.org/10.1093/bioinformatics/btp616

35. Tarazona S, García F, Ferrer A, Dopazo J, Conesa A (2012) NOIseq: a RNA-Seq differential expression method robust for sequencing depth biases. EMBnet J 17(B):18–19

36. Kim SK, Kim SY, Kim JH, Roh SA, Cho DH, Kim YS, Kim JC (2014) A nineteen gene-based risk score classifier predicts prognosis of colorectal cancer patients. Mol Oncol 8 (8):1653–1666. https://doi.org/10.1016/j.molonc.2014.06.016

37. Chatr-Aryamontri A, Breitkreutz BJ, Oughtred R, Boucher L, Heinicke S, Chen D, Stark C, Breitkreutz A, Kolas N, O'Donnell L, Reguly T, Nixon J, Ramage L, Winter A, Sellam A, Chang C, Hirschman J, Theesfeld C, Rust J, Livstone MS, Dolinski K, Tyers M (2015) The BioGRID interaction database: 2015 update. Nucleic Acids Res 43 (Database issue):D470–D478. https://doi.org/10.1093/nar/gku1204

38. Sales G, Calura E, Romualdi C (2012) GRAPH interaction from pathway topological environment BMC Bioinformatics 2013

39. Caspi R, Altman T, Billington R, Dreher K, Foerster H, Fulcher CA, Holland TA, Keseler IM, Kothari A, Kubo A, Krummenacker M, Latendresse M, Mueller LA, Ong Q, Paley S, Subhraveti P, Weaver DS, Weerasinghe D, Zhang P, Karp PD (2014) The MetaCyc database of metabolic pathways and enzymes and the BioCyc collection of Pathway/Genome Databases. Nucleic Acids Res 42(Database issue):D459–D471. https://doi.org/10.1093/nar/gkt1103

40. Mi H, Muruganujan A, Thomas PD (2013) PANTHER in 2013: modeling the evolution of gene function, and other gene attributes, in the context of phylogenetic trees. Nucleic Acids Res 41(Database issue):D377–D386. https://doi.org/10.1093/nar/gks1118

41. Schaefer CF, Anthony K, Krupa S, Buchoff J, Day M, Hannay T, Buetow KH (2009) PID: the Pathway Interaction Database. Nucleic Acids Res 37(Database issue):D674–D679. https://doi.org/10.1093/nar/gkn653

42. Gray KA, Yates B, Seal RL, Wright MW, Bruford EA (2015) Genenames.org: the HGNC resources in 2015. Nucleic Acids Res 43(Database issue):D1079–D1085. https://doi.org/10.1093/nar/gku1071

43. Maglott D, Ostell J, Pruitt KD, Tatusova T (2005) Entrez Gene: gene-centered information at NCBI. Nucleic Acids Res 33(Database issue):D54–D58. https://doi.org/10.1093/nar/gki031

44. Knijnenburg TA, Wessels LFA, Reinders MJT, Shmulevich I (2009) Fewer permutations, more accurate P-values. Bioinformatics 25 (12):i161–i168. https://doi.org/10.1093/bioinformatics/btp211

Chapter 4

QuickRNASeq: Guide for Pipeline Implementation and for Interactive Results Visualization

Wen He, Shanrong Zhao, Chi Zhang, Michael S. Vincent, and Baohong Zhang

Abstract

Sequencing of transcribed RNA molecules (RNA-Seq) has been used wildly for studying cell transcriptomes in bulk or at the single-cell level (Wang et al., Nat Rev Genet, 10:57–63, 2009; Ozsolak and Milos, Nat Rev Genet, 12:87–98, 2011; Sandberg, Nat Methods, 11:22–24, 2014) and is becoming the de facto technology for investigating gene expression level changes in various biological conditions, on the time course, and under drug treatments. Furthermore, RNA-Seq data helped identify fusion genes that are related to certain cancers (Maher et al., Nature, 458:97–101, 2009). Differential gene expression before and after drug treatments provides insights to mechanism of action, pharmacodynamics of the drugs, and safety concerns (Dixit et al., Genomics, 107:178–188, 2016). Because each RNA-Seq run generates tens to hundreds of millions of short reads with size ranging from 50 to 200 bp, a tool that deciphers these short reads to an integrated and digestible analysis report is in high demand. QuickRNASeq (Zhao et al., BMC Genomics, 17:39–53, 2016) is an application for large-scale RNA-Seq data analysis and real-time interactive visualization of complex data sets. This application automates the use of several of the best open-source tools to efficiently generate user friendly, easy to share, and ready to publish report. Figures in this protocol illustrate some of the interactive plots produced by QuickRNASeq. The visualization features of the application have been further improved since its first publication in early 2016. The original QuickRNASeq publication (Zhao et al., BMC Genomics, 17:39–53, 2016) provided details of background, software selection, and implementation. Here, we outline the steps required to implement QuickRNASeq in user's own environment, as well as demonstrate some basic yet powerful utilities of the advanced interactive visualization modules in the report.

Key words RNA-Seq, RNASeq, QuickRNASeq, RNA-Seq Pipeline, Transcriptome, Visualization, NGS data analysis

1 Introduction

Since its publication in early 2016, the QuickRNASeq pipeline has been adopted by many bioinformatics scientists and experimental researchers to do RNA-Seq data analysis, for its expedient

---

Wen He and Shanrong Zhao contributed equally to the manuscript.

Yejun Wang and Ming-an Sun (eds.), *Transcriptome Data Analysis: Methods and Protocols*, Methods in Molecular Biology, vol. 1751, https://doi.org/10.1007/978-1-4939-7710-9_4, © Springer Science+Business Media, LLC 2018

automation of the analysis pipeline and its convenient visualization. This detailed protocol provides instructions on installing every component of the pipeline, preparing sample data, running the pipeline for individual sequencing runs, merging results from different runs, interpreting the outcome and making figures for visualization. The goal of this protocol is to show you how to get the QucikRNASeq report from fastq files, as well as how to use the visualization features of the report. The structure of this protocol is outlined as follows. Subheading 2 is on Materials, and it describes the required hardware, software, and reference genome. Subheading 3 is on Methods. Subheading 3.1 describes the input files. Subheading 3.2 describes the command line call for individual runs. Subheading 3.3 is for combining the results from Subheading 3.2 to summary files and generating the report. Subheading 3.4 describes how to explore the report and make various plots from the interactive visualization tools. And finally, Subheading 4 includes notes for more productive use of QuickRNASeq.

2 Materials

2.1 Hardware

The QuickRNASeq package is fully tested on an HPC cluster using the IBM Platform LSF (Load Sharing Facility) or on a standalone workstation running Linux. Since the mapping step of millions of reads is a memory-demanding procedure, it is recommended to have 64GB per running instance. Other required hardware includes storage arrays with a high I/O throughput such as EMC Isilon if hundreds of samples are processed at the same time in parallel.

2.2 Software Prerequisites

Many open-source tools developed for RNA-Seq data analyses were tested before QuickRNASeq settled on the following five applications. STAR [7] was chosen for read alignment, or mapping, to reference genome and transcriptome assembly. FeatureCounts [8] from Subread package was adopted for counting reads to genomic features such as genes, exons, promoters, and genomic bins. VarScan [9] was used for variant calling. RSeQC [10] was chosen for RNA-Seq quality control. Samtools [11] provides various utilities for manipulating alignments in the SAM format. These open source tools should be installed as instructed below. Names of directories are for demonstration only, which should be replaced by your own names.

2.2.1 STAR

Download STAR from https://github.com/alexdobin/STAR/releases.
Install STAR to /opt/ngsapp/STAR_2.4.0 k/bin/Linux_x86_64.

2.2.2 Subread

Download Subread packages from http://subread.sourceforge.net/.
Install Subread to /opt/ngsapp/subread-1.4.6/bin.

2.2.3 VarScan	Download JAR file from http://varscan.sourceforge.net/. Install VarScan to /opt/ngsapp/bin/VarScan.v2.4.0.jar.
2.2.4 RSeQC	Download and install RSeQC from http://rseqc.sourceforge.net/. Install RSeQC to /opt/ngsapp/anaconda/bin.
2.2.5 Samtools	Download Samtools from http://sourceforge.net/projects/samtools/files/. Install Samtools to /opt/ngsapp/bin.

2.3 Download QuickRNASeq Package

QuickRNASeq [6] is available from sourceforge. Follow this link to download the source code: https://sourceforge.net/projects/quickrnaseq. The protocol is based on version 1.2.

We have QuickRNASeq installed at directory /opt/ngsapp/QuickRNASeq.

2.4 Preparation of Genome Fasta File, Annotation, and Index

Here we show how to create the index for RNA-Seq analysis using Gencode release 23 of human genome GRCh38 as an example. For details of STAR related command line parameters, please refer to recent publication from Dobin and Gingeras on optimizing RNA-Seq mapping with STAR [12].

1. Download genome fasta file
   ftp://ftp.sanger.ac.uk/pub/gencode/Gencode_human/release_23/GRCh38.primary_assembly.genome.fa.gz.

2. Download gene annotation in GTF format
   ftp://ftp.sanger.ac.uk/pub/gencode/Gencode_human/release_23/gencode.v23.annotation.gtf.gz.

3. Unzip and rename genome and GTF file
   Unzip and rename genome fasta file and GTF file as GRCh38.primary.genome.fa, GRCh38.gencode.v23.gtf respectively. Save these two files in the corresponding project data folder. In this example, genome fasta file is saved to directory /opt/fasta; GTF annotation file to directory /opt/gencode

4. Prepare annotation and BED files using utility functions in QuickRNASeq
   Make sure you are in directory /opt/gencode, and call QuickRNASeq utility functions as shown below:

```
/opt/ngsapp/QuickRNASeq/gtf2bed.pl GRCh38.gencode.v23.gtf >
GRCh38.gencode.v23.bed
/opt/ngsapp/QuickRNASeq/gtf2annot.pl GRCh38.gencode.v23.gtf >
GRCh38.gencode.v23.annot
/opt/ngsapp/bin/samtools faidx GRCh38.primary.genome.fa
```

5. Create genome index file
   In this example, we are creating a genome index for read length up to 100 bp. Under directory /opt/STAR/, create a directory

called GRCh38_gencode23_100. Move to this GRCh38_gen-code23_100 directory, and create genome index as shown below. The option sjdbOverhang is set at 99. In general, sjdbO-verhang is set as "read length - 1". An example command is listed below:

```
/opt/ngsapp/STAR_2.4.0k/bin/Linux_x86_64/STAR  --runThreadN
32 --runMode
genomeGenerate --genomeDir
/opt/STAR/GRCh38_gencode23_100 -genomeFastaFiles /opt/fasta/
GRCh38.primary.genome.fa -sjdbGTFfile
/opt/gencode/GRCh38.gencode.v23.gtf --sjdbOverhang 99
```

6. Find the chromosome where MHC genes are located
   MHC genes are highly polymorphic, which makes this region ideal for checking sample SNP concordance. In the human genome, the MHC region occurs on chromosome 6. Get the corresponding coordinate for chromosome 6 from chrName-Length.txt file in the STAR index result folder. In this case, the coordinate is 1–170805979.

   After the above steps are completed, you are ready to set the reference genome related parameters in the configuration file. Refer to Subheading 3.1.3, **step 6** for instructions.

3   Methods

The QuickRNASeq pipeline can be divided into the following three main steps:

1. Prepare RNA-Seq input data, including a sample configuration file.
2. Process individual samples, including mapping, counting, and QC.
3. Merge results from individual sample and generate an integrated report.

The first step is specific to individual runs and samples within those runs. This step needs to be tailored for each RNA-Seq run. The last step is more or less fixed. A master-cmd.sh file included in the package contains the common commands to be called for step 2 and step 3. Nevertheless, all environmental variables need to be set correctly to ensure the scripts in master-cmd.sh will work well. All these steps should be performed under a project folder for all samples belonging to a specific project.

After downloading QucikRNASeq1.2, you will see a directory named "test_run". This is an example project directory. We are using the same 48 GTEx samples from 5 donors as in the original

QuickRNASeq publication [6]. This test_run project directory contains key files for running QuickRNASeq. The following discussions describe the contents of these files, and step-by-step instructions to guide you through the process.

3.1 Prepare RNA-Seq Input Data

3.1.1 Prepare a Sample Annotation File and a Sample ID File

1. Annotation file
   To run QuickRNASeq, a user needs to provide meaningful annotations for all samples. A proper annotation file should be in tab delimited text *see* **Note 1**. The first and second columns correspond to sample and subject identifiers, respectively. Although not required, it is highly recommended to use "sample_id" and "subject_id" for the first two columns while the rest of the columns are flexible, based on project design. The sample. annotation.txt file in test_run directory has columns as "Run", "subject_id", "histological_type", and "sex".

2. Sample ID file
   Sample ID file contains one unique sample ID per line. There is no column header. The allIDs.txt file in test_run directory lists all 48 samples in this demo project. For example, the first sample ID is "SRR607214".

3.1.2 Prepare Fastq Files for each Individual Sample

For paired end sequencing, prepare two fastq files, one for each read. Format will be sample_id_1.fastq.gz and sample_id_2.fastq. gz. For example, sample SRR607214 will have two files: SRR607214_1.fastq.gz, and SRR607214_2.fastq.gz.

Some new Illumina sequencing platforms, such as Next-Seq500, generate eight files as output for each sample in paired end sequencing. In this case, we need to concatenate these fastq files into two files, one for each read of paired end sequencing. Make sure the concatenation order is the same for both files.

There will be only one fastq file per sample if the sequence run is single end.

At the end of this step, we will have "N" numbers of fastq files if the run contains "N" single read samples. Or we have "$2 \times N$" of fastq files if the sequencing is paired end run. We save these files in a directory called fastq.

3.1.3 Set Up Run Configuration File

File run.config is a project-specific configuration file that contains all sequencing, genome, and software related information for QuickRNASeq analysis. Genome and software portions only need to be changed if there are updates on tools or alterations on genome, index and/or annotation. The sequencing run-specific portion is what we need to modify for each analysis. Please refer to $QuickRNASeq/star-fc-qc.config.template for more details. You can copy star-fc-qc.config.template in QuickRNASeq package to your project folder and then customize it to your environment. Please see directory test_run for an example of run.config file.

1. Set FASTQ_DIR:
   FASTQ_DIR is the directory where the fastq files are located. You can set a fastq directory within the project folder to store all fastq files, or you can store your fastq file in another location.

2. Set the suffix for fastq file:
   QuickRNASeq will automatically add "_1. FASTQ_SUFFIX" and "_2. FASTQ_SUFFIX" to each sample ID in the allID.txt file, and look for these files in the FASTQ_DIR. The name of the fastq file should match the name in the allID.txt file. For example, for sample SRR607214, if you set FASTQ_SUFFIX = fastq. gz, the program will go to directory FASTQ_DIR and look files SRR607214_1.fastq.gz and SRR607214_2.fastq.gz. Sometimes, the fastq files end as fq.gz, sometimes, it ends as fastq. gz. In our example run.config file, it was set as FASTQ_SUFFIX = fastq.gz.

3. Set strand information:
   STRAND=0 for nonstranded RNA-Seq.
   STRAND=1 for first read forward strand.
   STRAND=2 for first read reverse strand, for instance Illumina's sequencing kit

4. Set sequencing depth:
   There are two choices for sequencing depth option. Set it to "regular" if the sequencing run generates 40–80 million reads; or set it to "deep" if the run generates 100 million reads or more. For example: SEQUENCE_DEPTH = regular.

5. Set sequence type:
   This is to state whether your read is paired or single (e.g., SEQUENCE_TYPE = pair).

6. Set species-specific genome index and GTF file:
   These options will not change unless the genome reference changes. Please refer to Subheading 2.4 for instruction on how to generate these species-specific files.

```
GENOME_FASTA=/opt/fasta/GRCh38.primary.genome.fa
GENOME_INDEX=/opt/STAR/GRCh38_gencode23_100
GENOME_ANNOTATION=/opt/gencode/GRCh38.gencode.v23.annot
GTF_FILE=/opt/gencode/GRCh38.gencode.v23.gtf
BEDFILE=/opt/gencode/GRCh38.gencode.v23.bed
CHR_REGION=chr6:1-170805979
```

7. Set the environmental variables for tools installed at Subheading 2.2:

   Software locations will remain the same unless there is a major update.

```
STAR_RNA=/opt/ngsapp/STAR_2.4.0k/bin/Linux_x86_64
FEATURECOUNTS=/opt/ngsapp/subread-1.4.6/bin
RSeQC=/opt/ngsapp/anaconda/bin
```

```
VARSCAN_JAR=/opt/ngsapp/bin/VarScan.v2.4.0.jar
SAMTOOLS=/opt/ngsapp/bin
```

3.2 Run the QuickRNASeq Script to Process Individual Samples

QuickRNASeq calls R and Rscript. Please make sure R version 3.1 or above and these R packages, ggplot2, edgeR, scales, and reshape2 are installed on your machine.

Under your project folder, invoke mapping, counting, QC, and SNP call for each sample by calling star-fc-qc.sh. Make sure that the $PATH environmental variable includes the path to QuickRNA-Seq_1.2 location. Because this step is computationally intensive, it is advised to run this command on HPC clusters using LSF as a job scheduler. A separate result folder will be created for each sample under the project folder. In addition to LSF, there is a list of notable job scheduling software available to choose from. For a cluster using a job scheduler other than LSF, star-fc-qc.sh needs to be twisted or modified. For people who have no access to a HPC cluster, we offer star-fc-qc.ws.sh, a customized script working in a standard Linux workstation. Of course, analyzing a large RNA-Seq dataset in a single workstation is not typical. Below is the command call example.

```
# ENVIRONMENT
export QuickRNASeq={QuickRNASeq_installation_Directory}
# e.g. export QuickRNASeq=/opt/ngsapp/QuickRNASeq_1.2
export PATH=$QuickRNASeq:$PATH
star-fc-qc.sh allIDs.txt run.config

#run the following command if you run the analysis on a
standalone workstation
#star-fc-qc.ws.sh allIDs.txt run.config
```

3.3 Merge Results from Individual Samples and Generate an Integrated Report

As in the previous steps, this step also runs under the project directory. We run the merging and summarization step when all jobs are finished for each sample. The sample.annotation.txt should include all samples to be merged. Each sample has to be processed as listed in Subheading 3.2. Below are commands to run in order to generate the report. "GENE_ANNOTATION" points to a file containing gene descriptions that can be obtained by running "Rscript $QuickRNASeq /QuickRNASeq_html/getEnsemblAnno.R".

```
#Summarization, only run it when all jobs are finished in the
first step
export GENOME_ANNOTATION=/opt/gencode/hg19.gencode.v19.annot
export GENE_ANNOTATION=/opt/gencode/Ensembl_v75_hg19_Gen-
code.v19_human.txt.gz
nohup star-fc-qc.summary.sh sample.annotation.txt &> Re-
```

```
sults.log
#run the command line below if you run the analysis in a
workstation
#star-fc.summary.sh sample.annotation.txt
```

3.3.1 QuickRNASeq Test Run

We made a test run available for you to test the QuickRNASeq software before applying this tool to your data. Adjust QuickRNA-Seq to point to your QuickRNASeq installation folder. Please refer to $QuickRNASeq/test_run folder for:

- allIDs.txt: sample identifiers.
- sample.annotation.txt: annotation file.
- run.config: sample configuration file.
- master-cmd.sh: command lines for test runs. Please run step #2 after step #1 finishes.

3.3.2 Description of Output Files

The output of the merge command is a directory called Results. Seven html files (gex.html, index.html*, longitudinal.html, qc_fc-counting-summary.html, qc_expr_count_RPKM.html, qc_over-view.html, qc_star-mapping-summary.html) and three directories (package, QC, summary) will be generated within the Results directory.

This Results directory can be copied to your laptop or desktop. Open index.html within Results directory to access the interactive report in html format. Alternatively, this Results directory can be hosted on a web server to share with other group members, which also makes this QuickRNASeq report available at all times. Summary directory contains all summary files which are displayed on the html report under the "Raw Data Files" section.

3.4 Explore Integrated and Interactive Report

Open the index.html file under Results directory and you will have access to all data and figures. You will be able to drill down RNA-Seq analysis results in an interactive way. We implemented the interactive data visualization in QuickRNASeq using these JavaScript-based open-source libraries including JQuery [13], D3 (Data-Driven Documents) [14], canvasXpress [15], SlickGrid [16], and Nozzle [17]. The figures and tables in QC Metrics and QC Plot portion of the QuickRNASeq web report have been introduced and described in the original publication [6]. Some of these figures are showcased in Fig. 1. Below, we focus on the interactive plotting features that can be accessed by clicking the pointing hand next to "RPKM Values on Genes" under the Expression Table section.

3.4.1 Meaning of Mouse Icons

Pointing hand, click to get interactive plot. Left click; Right click; Double left click; Scroll middle wheel.

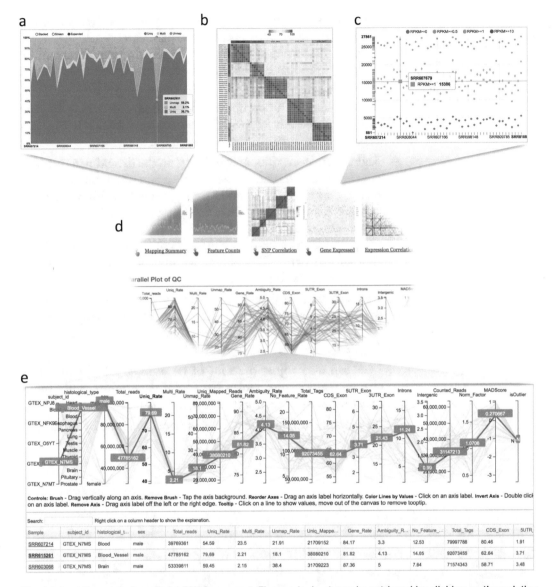

Fig. 1 Interactive plots from QuickRNASeq report. Figures (a, b, c) can be retrieved by clicking on the pointing hands as shown in Fig. 1d. On any of these interactive plots, mouse over each sample displays associated sample QC metrics. (**a**) Read mapping summary in the expanded display mode. (**b**) SNP concordance matrix of 48 samples from 5 donors. Samples from the same donor should be highly concordant. (**c**) Gene expression chart, which shows the number of genes past various expression thresholds. (**d**) Center portion of the QuickRNASeq report. (**e**) Parallel plot linking multiple QC measures for the same samples plus table of multidimensional QC measures

3.4.2 Create a Boxplot for One Gene

1. Figure 2 combines six charts to demonstrate how to create a boxplot for gene expression of a single gene. From the main QuickRNASeq report HTML page, click on the 👆 "pointing hand" icon in the Expression Table section to get to gene expression Table. A new HTML page will show up, *see* Fig. 2a.

This webpage is from file gex.html, which was generated as a result of running star-fc-qc.summary.sh.

2. Search by keyword and then left click on any column except the first two on a gene (Fig. 2a). As demonstrated in Fig. 2a, we searched by "kinase", then selected gene "CAMKK1".

3. A new window pops up which displays a dot plot of gene expression level in RPKM value for kinase CAMKK1 (Fig. 2b). Please note that the X-axis is smaple ID.

4. Right click on any plot area to bring up the drop down menu for sample grouping, data transformation and chart customization. As shown in Fig. 2c, samples were grouped by following menu "Group Samples" and then "histological_type" for box plot. Please note that in Fig. 2c, X-axis is histological_type. Click on any plot area to hide the menu and you should see the boxplot (not shown here). The sample features are gathered from the "sample.annotation.txt" file.

5. Data can be transformed to various scales by right clicking on the plot to bring up the menu and then following "Data" ->"Transform" ->"Log Base 2" for log2 transformation (Fig. 2d).

6. User can also adjust the font of the sample label, add Y-axis, change window and canvas size, color data points, and explore many other visualization features, see Note 2.

7. Data points can be connected as shown in Fig. 2e by subject_id.

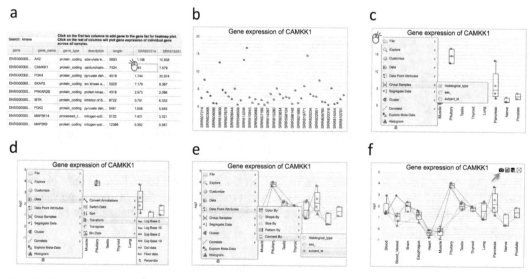

Fig. 2 Boxplot of a gene. (**a**) From gene expression table, search genes by keyword "kinase," and select gene CAMKK1. (**b**) Dot plot of CAMKK1 gene expression across all samples. (**c**) Group sample by histological type. (**d**) Log2 transformation of expression level. (**e**) Connect data point by subject identifier. (**f**) Take the screenshot of the boxplot as a png image

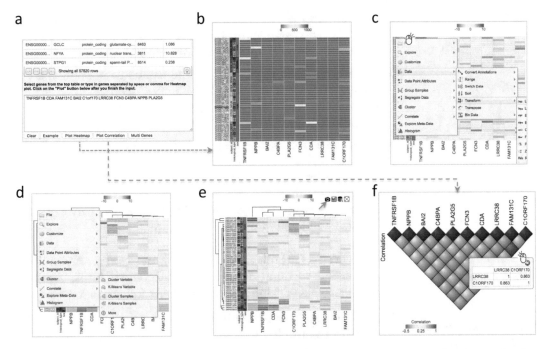

Fig. 3 Generation of heatmap for a list of genes. (**a**) Select from the above table or enter a list of genes into the text box. (**b**) Initial heatmap. (**c**) Log2 transformation of expression level. (**d**) Cluster samples and variables. (**e**) A final heatmap ready to be saved in png format. (**f**) Gene expression correlation plot

8. When you are satisfied with the settings, move mouse up to the top of the canvas to activate the top menu, where you will see a "Camera" icon. Click on the "Camera" icon to get a screenshot in png format for publication (Fig. 2f).

3.4.3 Create a Heatmap for Multiple Genes

1. Figure 3 consists of several charts which illustrate the steps involved for drawing a gene expression heatmap. As shown in Fig. 3a, in the large text box below the table of expression, there are ten genes, which are "TNFRSF1B CDA FAM131C BAI2 C1orf170 LRRC38 FCN3 C4BPA NPPB PLA2G5". These genes can be typed in the text box, or select one by one from the expression table above the text box. You can also copy and paste the gene list separated by space or comma. Copying and pasting the gene list from an Excel file also works. It is suggested to enter the official HUGO gene symbol for each gene. After you have the gene list, click on "Plot Heatmap" button, a heatmap shows up, as in Fig. 3b.

2. Expression level from different genes could vary widely. It is a good idea to have the heatmap displays gene expression level in log2 format. Right click on any plot area to bring up the drop down menu for data transformation. The example in Fig. 3c is transforming data into Log Base 2.

3. Cluster samples by following menu "Cluster" ->"Cluster Samples". Cluster variables by following menu "Cluster" ->"Cluster Variables". *See* Fig. 3d for a demonstration.

4. Move mouse up to the top of the canvas to activate the top menu, where you will see the "Camera" icon again, and then click on the "Camera" icon to get a png image ready for publication (Fig. 3e).

5. Figure 3f is for expression correlation among the genes in the gene list. Click "Plot Correlation" to get the correlation picture shown in Fig. 3f. Double clicking on any square will show the correlation value between two genes. The example in Fig. 3f shows the expression correlation across samples between gene LRRC38 and gene C1ORF170 is 0.863.

3.5 Make the Report Publicly Available at github.com

You will need a GitHub account to perform this step. If you don't have a GitHub account, create one first by going to https://github.com. To create a GitHub repository, please follow these two steps.

3.5.1 Create a Repository by Login github.com

1. Click on the "New repository" icon as shown in Fig. 4a after GitHub account login.

2. Type in project name and description and then click "Create repository" icon as illustrated in Fig. 4b. Please use your own project name instead of "RNASeq_1" that is for illustration purpose only.

3.5.2 Commands to Publish the Report Files to GitHub Repository

Change texts in red to your own settings.

git clone https://github.com/username/RNASeq_1.git

cd RNASeq_1

git checkout --orphan gh-pages

cp -R path2result/Results/* .

git add .

git commit -a -m "Adding RNASeq_1 results from QuickRNASeq"

git push origin gh-pages

Now, the report should be available at http://username.github.io/RNASeq_1

The demo page for the example data set is at http://baohongz.github.io/QuickRNASeq

4 Notes

1. Wired Characters in Input Files

a

b

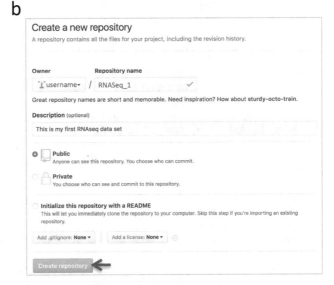

Fig. 4 Creation of a GitHub repository. (**a**) Repository panel is located on the right side of the web page after GitHub login. The red arrow points to the "New repository" button. (**b**) Fill in "Repository name" field using your own name and check the "Public" radio button if you want to publish it to the Internet then click "Create repository" to finish

Although we have taken multiple measures to either remove or replace R unfriendly characters and unnecessary blank spaces in user input files such as sample.annotation.txt, it is recommended to use only alphanumeric and tab characters in these files. If Microsoft Excel is used to create the sample.annotation.txt, please make sure that you save it in tab-delimited format

2. Further customization of plots

   (a) The font of sample labels will be enlarged by following "Customize" ->"Sample Labels" ->"Font" ->"Bigger". The more you click on the "Bigger" button, the larger the font becomes.

   (b) Add y-axis title by following "Customize" ->"Axes Titles" ->"Text". Type in title in the input box and then click the nearby cycling button.

   (c) The size of Pop-up Window and Canvas can be altered by click-and-drag the left bottom corner as indicated by the black arrow that will appear while the mouse moves over.

   (d) Follow "Data Points Attributes" ->"Color by" to color data points based on certain feature.

References

1. Wang Z, Gerstein M, Snyder M (2009) RNA-Seq: a revolutionary tool for transcriptomics. Nat Rev Genet 10(1):57–63

2. Ozsolak F, Milos PM (2011) RNA sequencing: advances, challenges and opportunities. Nat Rev Genet 12:87–98

3. Sandberg R (2014) Entering the era of single-cell transcriptomics in biology and medicine. Nat Methods 11:22–24

4. Maher CA, Kumar-Sinha C, Cao X, Kalyana-Sundaram S, Han B, Jing X, Sam L, Barrette T, Palanisamy N, Chinnaiyan AM (2009) Transcriptome sequencing to detect gene fusions in cancer. Nature 458(7234):97–101

5. Dixit AB, Banerjee J, Srivastava A, Tripathi M, Sarkar C, Kakkar A, Jain M, Chandra PS (2016) RNA-Seq analysis of hippocampal tissues reveals novel candidate genes for drug refractory epilepsy in patients with MTLE-HS. Genomics 107(5):178–188

6. Zhao S, Xi L, Jie Q, Xi H, Zhang Y, von Schack D, Vincent M, Zhang B (2016) QuickRNASeq lifts large-scale RNA-Seq data analyses to the next level of automation and interactive visualization. BMC Genomics 17:39–53

7. Dobin A, Davis CA, Schlesinger F, Drenkow J, Zaleski C, Jha S et al (2013) STAR: ultrafast universal RNA-Seq aligner. Bioinformatics 29(1):15–21

8. Liao Y, Smyth GK, Shi W (2014) feature-Counts: an efficient general purpose program for assigning sequence reads to genomic features. Bioinformatics 30(7):923–930

9. Koboldt D, Zhang Q, Larson D, Shen D, McLellan M, Lin L et al (2012) VarScan 2: somatic mutation and copy number alteration discovery in cancer by exome sequencing. Genome Res 22:568–576

10. Wang L, Wang S, Li W (2012) RSeQC: quality control of RNA-Seq experiments. Bioinformatics 28(16):2184–2185

11. Li H, Handsaker B, Wysoker A, Fennell T, Ruan J, Homer N, Marth G, Abecasis G, Durbin R, 1000 Genome Project Data Processing Subgroup (2009) The sequence alignment/map (SAM) format and SAMtools. Bioinformatics 25:2078–2079

12. Dobin A, Gngeras TR (2016) Optimizing RNA-Seq mapping with STAR. In: Carugo O, Eisenhaber F (eds) Data mining techniques for the life sciences, methods in molecular biology, vol 1415. Springer Science+Business Media, New York

13. jQuery. https://jquery.com. Accessed 15 Nov 2015

14. Data-Driven Documents. http://d3js.org. Accessed 15 Nov 2015

15. canvasXpress. http://canvasxpress.org. Accessed 15 Nov 2015

16. SlickGrid. https://github.com/mleibman/SlickGrid. Accessed 15 Nov 2015

17. Gehlenborg N, Noble MS, Getz G, Chin L, Park PJ (2013) Nozzle: a report generation toolkit for data analysis pipelines. Bioinformatics 29:1089–1091

Part II

Objective-Specialized Transcriptome Data Analysis

Chapter 5

Tracking Alternatively Spliced Isoforms from Long Reads by SpliceHunter

Zheng Kuang and Stefan Canzar

Abstract

Alternative splicing increases the functional complexity of a genome by generating multiple isoforms and potentially proteins from the same gene. Vast amounts of alternative splicing events are routinely detected by short read deep sequencing technologies but their functional interpretation is hampered by an uncertain transcript context. Emerging long-read sequencing technologies provide a more complete picture of full-length transcript sequences. We introduce SpliceHunter, a tool for the computational interpretation of long reads generated by for example Pacific Biosciences instruments. SpliceHunter defines and tracks isoforms and novel transcription units across time points, compares their splicing pattern to a reference annotation, and translates them into potential protein sequences.

Key words Alternative splicing, PacBio sequencing, RNA sequencing, Transcript isoform, Long-read sequencing, SpliceHunter, Time course analysis

1 Introduction

Alternative splicing (AS) is an important mechanism of gene expression regulation that allows to generate multiple transcript variants (isoforms) from the same gene, through selective usage of exons and their splice sites [1]. AS is prevalent across different cell types and different conditions. For example, AS occurs in >90% of multiexon genes in major human tissues [2, 3]. However, the extent and the biological meaning are still not well understood. A major limitation of second generation sequencing technology is the local information content of short read sequences that allow to detect individual AS events but fail to provide the global picture of full-length transcript sequences, which impedes the understanding of the functional consequences of AS. Third generation sequencing by for example Pacific Biosciences (PacBio) SMRT technology [4], generates multikilobases long reads and thus valuable data for the detection of full-length transcripts. We have developed the computational tool SpliceHunter to interpret these

Yejun Wang and Ming-an Sun (eds.), *Transcriptome Data Analysis: Methods and Protocols*, Methods in Molecular Biology, vol. 1751, https://doi.org/10.1007/978-1-4939-7710-9_5, © Springer Science+Business Media, LLC 2018

long-read data and characterize the structure and dynamic abundance of isoforms. SpliceHunter has previously been used to characterize the diversity and the dynamics of isoforms expressed during the meiosis of fission yeast [5]. It tracks and compares isoforms across time points (e.g., in meiosis), cell types, or conditions.

In contrast to widely used short read analysis methods like MISO [6], MATS [7], JuncBase [8], and JUM [9] that statistically compare the usage of (individual) splice junctions, we have developed SpliceHunter to support the explorative analysis of long sequencing reads produced by third generation technology like PacBio and Oxford nanopore [10]. SpliceHunter defines and tracks full length isoforms across time points (or conditions in general) and annotates their molecularly phased AS by comparing them to an existing annotation. It applies precisely defined criteria to uniquely label AS events as exon skipping, intron retention, their counterparts exon inclusions and introns in exons, respectively, alternative acceptors and donors, and novel exons.

It further provides dimer or hexamer sequences and the length distribution of novel, annotated or retained introns for downstream analysis of splicing preferences. More importantly, the interpretation of long reads is not affected by the uncertainty that lies in the isoform assemblies computed by methods like Cufflinks [11] and CIDANE [12] from short reads, but SpliceHunter simply clusters compatible long reads to isoforms. This facilitates the study of molecular coassociation of splicing events as well as functional consequences of AS. For the former, SpliceHunter counts reads that support pairs of AS events and the constituent singletons. For the latter, SpliceHunter translates RNA sequences of isoforms into protein sequences that can be used to investigate the conservation across species or to study the impact of AS on the protein's (predicted [13]) secondary or tertiary structure.

We provide tailored R code [14] to transform SpliceHunter's text-based output into statistics and visual illustrations of the AS landscape, the exon–intron structure of inferred isoforms, the dynamic changes of isoform abundances, as well as a statistical evaluation of coassociation of AS events.

Long-read sequencing technology combined with tailored methods like SpliceHunter will open a big window to isoform-level RNA biology.

2   Materials

2.1   Hardware

SpliceHunter has been developed and tested on a 64-bit Linux (x86_64) and Mac OS X system.

The amount of main memory (RAM) it requires depends on the size of the genome and the complexity of the transcriptome. While it uses only around 100 MB of RAM to analyse the transcriptome of the unicellular model organism *Schizosacccharo-myces pombe*, we recommend at least 4 GB of RAM for more complex organisms.

The FASTA/FASTQ files containing the reference genome sequence and the raw reads as well as read alignments in SAM/-BAM format typically require moderate to large disc space (>10GB), depending on the experiment.

2.2 Software

SpliceHunter is free open-source software released under the GNU GPL license and is available at https://bitbucket.org/canzar/splicehunter. SpliceHunter can be built from source code with the CMake build system, for which we provide a step-by-step guide on the bitbucket website. Alternatively, precompiled executables for Linux and Mac OS X are available in the Downloads section of the website. SpliceHunter depends on libraries SeqAn, Boost, and zlib, and has been bundled with BamTools to simplify the installation process. Instructions on where to obtain these libraries can be found on the website. Before running SpliceHunter, raw reads need to be classified as (non) full-length and clustered using the Iso-Seq protocol [15] and mapped to the reference genome using GMAP [16]:

The isoform sequencing (Iso-Seq) pipeline can be run in a browser through the SMRT Portal. A more detailed instruction can be found in the RNA sequencing subsection of the SMRT Portal   http://www.pacb.com/products-and-services/analytical-software/smrt-analysis/.

The genomic origin of mRNA reads is determined by aligning them to the reference sequence across introns using GMAP. The latest release of GMAP as well as a manual on its use is available at http://research-pub.gene.com/gmap/. Alternatively, GMAP can be run directly through the SMRT Portal.

The output of SpliceHunter is further processed, analyzed, and visually summarized in R. We provide the necessary R code as well as a shell script to produce .bam files for the visualization of isoform dynamics in IGV [17] (*see* Subheading 3.4, **step 7**) in subdirectory scripts/.

2.3 Input Files

The reference transcriptome to which inferred isoforms are structurally compared is read from an annotation file in GFF/GTF format. The reference genome sequence must be provided in FASTA format. Raw reads are expected in FASTQ or FASTA format.

Example data used in this tutorial, including reference sequence, transcriptome, and PacBio reads, are available for download at LRZ Sync+Share [18].

We use the first replicate of the time-course PacBio sequencing data from our previous study [5] to illustrate how to detect, annotate, and track isoforms with SpliceHunter and how to process and interpret its results. The data were sampled every 2 h from 0 to 10 h during the meiosis of *S. pombe*.

3   Methods

The complete workflow from data preprocessing to the tracking of isoforms with SpliceHunter and the final visualization in R is shown in Fig. 1.

3.1   Preprocessing

The Iso-Seq pipeline is composed of two major modules: The classify module identifies full-length and non-full-length transcript reads based on the presence of 5′ and 3′ cDNA primer sequences

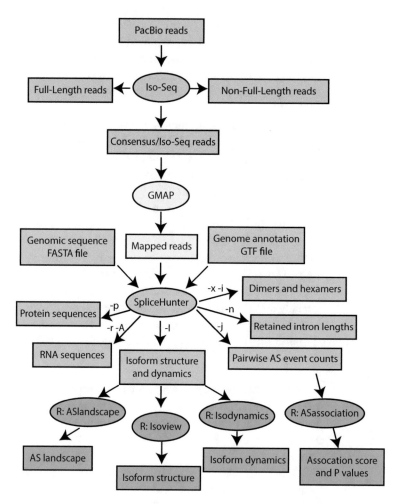

Fig. 1 The workflow of isoform analysis. It consists of four major steps: orange: Iso-Seq preprocessing of reads into consensus isoforms ("Iso-Seq reads"), yellow: mapping Iso-Seq reads to the reference sequence with GMAP, green: isoform detection with SpliceHunter, and blue: downstream analysis and visualization in R and IGV. Arrow labels indicate SpliceHunter options that control the corresponding output

and the polyA/polyT sequence. The cluster module generates preliminary consensus isoforms using full-length reads and uses non-full-length reads to polish the consensus sequences. The SMRT Portal integrates the two modules in one step and allows to run the Iso-Seq protocol as follows:

1. Create a new job and select the Iso-Seq protocol named "RS_IsoSeq.1".

2. Use default values for Minimum Full Passes (0) and Minimum Predicted Accuracy (75) at the filtering step or adjust if necessary.

3. Use default value of 300 for Minimum Sequence Length at the Isoseq_classify step or adjust accordingly. Make sure to unselect the "Full-length Reads Do Not Require PolyA Tails."

4. Select "Predict Consensus Isoforms Using The ICE Algorithm" and "Call Quiver To Polish Concensus Isoforms" at the Isoseq_cluster step. Select the correct cDNA Size setting based on the library size.

5. After the analysis has completed, download the cluster fasta file. FASTA files containing the predicted consensus isoforms are recommended for downstream analysis. For high quality purposes, Quiver Polished High QV consensus isoform FASTA files can be used.

3.2 Mapping

We use GMAP to map the consensus sequences (henceforth referred to as Iso-Seq reads) to the reference genome. Although GMAP is available through the SMRT Portal, we recommend downloading and running the latest version manually. To align the reads in our sample data using 4 threads, run:

```
gmap -d pombe -D pombe_1225/pombe -t 4 -n 0 -f samse
ZK1_all_isoforms.fasta > b1_151204_1.sam
```

This returns the alignments in SAM format (-f samse). The SAM alignemnt file can be converted to a more compact BAM file required by SpliceHunter:

```
samtools view -bS b1_151204_1.sam > b1_151204_1.bam
```

For visualization of the alignments in IGV, the BAM file needs to be sorted and indexed:

```
samtools sort b1_151204_1.bam b1_151204_1.sort.bam
samtools index b1_151204_1.sort.bam
```

3.3 SpliceHunter

SpliceHunter infers complex splicing patterns along novel isoforms in three main steps. After assigning reads to known genes or novel transcription units, reads are clustered to isoforms based on a consistent splicing pattern. Each isoform is then compared one-by-one to the reference transcripts of the assigned gene to annotate its sequence of alternative splicing events. Finally, SpliceHunter writes the full RNA sequence of isoforms and novel TUs as well as their putative protein sequences to FASTA files, which can be used (by, e.g., BLAST [19]) to study conservation across related species on the protein level. SpliceHunter's behavior in each step can be controlled by different options (see arrow labels in Fig. 1) and is explained in more detail below.

SpliceHunter can be run from the command line as follows:

```
SpliceHunter [options]* --gtf <reference_annotation.gtf> -f
<genome_sequence.fa> -m <bam_directory>
```

SpliceHunter writes all detected and annotated isoforms as well as TUs to the console ("standard out") by default. Ambiguous reads, among which potentially inter-strand fused RNA molecules lie, are reported in ambiguous.txt.

3.3.1 Main Arguments

```
-g/--gtf <reference_annotation.gtf>
```

SpliceHunter compares all isoforms detected from the read data to annotated gene structures provided by this reference annotation in GTF format.

```
-f/--ref <genome_sequence.fa>
```

SpliceHunter looks up sequence information in the supplied FASTA file.

```
-m/--dir
```

SpliceHunter will jointly analyze all read alignment files (.bam) it finds in the specified directory. It will interpret file names as <replicate>_*_<condition>.bam, where samples are collected across different conditions or time points and grouped as replicates.

```
-I/--iso <isoform_file.txt>
```

SpliceHunter writes all detected and annotated isoforms to file <isoform_file.txt>. By default, SpliceHunter prints isoforms to the "standard out" file handle, that is, to the console.

3.3.2 Data Preprocessing

To increase confidence that a read alignment represents the true origin of the read and that the read is correctly split across introns, SpliceHunter applies additional quality requirements that can be adjusted as follows:

`-a/--maplength <float>`

SpliceHunter ignores read mappings with less than a fraction of `<float>` of its bases aligned ('M' in CIGAR string). Default: 0.67.

`-q/--mapqual <float>`

SpliceHunter ignores read mappings with less than a fraction of `<float>` of its aligned bases ('M' in CIGAR string) being identical to the reference base. Default: 0.75.

`-e/--ewin <int>`

SpliceHunter discards reads which align with a mismatch or indel within `<int>` bases of at least one of its implied novel splice sites, unless it can rescue the novel splice site (`--swin`). Default: 10 bp.

`-w/--swin <int>`

SpliceHunter discards reads which align with a mismatch or indel close to (`--ewin`) one of its splice sites, unless it can shift the formerly novel splice site to an annotated splice site located within `<int>` bases. Default: 10 bp.

SpliceHunter keeps track of the number of CCS reads supporting all Iso-Seq reads contained in an isoform cluster. It counts both full length (FL) CCS reads and non-FL CCS reads associated with an Iso-Seq read, whose number it derives from the read's identifier (i.e., QNAME in .bam file). In particular, Iso-Seq assigns reads ids following the format `*/f<x>p<y>/*`, where `<x>` denotes the number of full length CCS reads, and `<y>` the number of non-FL CCS reads. Optionally, SpliceHunter can rely on FL CCS reads only:

`-1/--fl`

SpliceHunter counts only full length (FL) CCS reads supporting an Iso-Seq read and ignores all other reads (non-FL CCS) in the analysis.

3.3.3 Gene Assignment

SpliceHunter first tries to assign a spliced read alignment to an annotated gene on either strand by an exact match of any of its introns. If the read's introns match at least one intron of one annotated gene only, the read is assigned to that gene. If the read's introns match introns of multiple annotated genes on the same strand, SpliceHunter outputs the read as a read-through transcripts, and as an interstrand fused RNA molecule if these genes are located on different strands. If none of the read's introns matches any annotated intron, SpliceHunter examines individual splice sites for an exact match in the annotation. More precisely, every "left" (i.e., smaller coordinate) splice site of a read intron is searched for a matching annotated donor site on the forward strand or annotated acceptor site on the reverse strand. Similarly, every "right" (i.e., larger coordinate) splice site of a read intron is searched for a matching annotated acceptor site on the forward strand or annotated donor site on the reverse strand. If the read's splice sites match at least one splice site of one gene only, the read is assigned to that gene. If they match the splice sites of multiple genes, the read is output as ambiguous and ignored in further analysis. If no matching splice site was found either, SpliceHunter attempts to assign the read to an annotated gene by exonic overlap. If the exons of a read overlap with the exons of one annotated gene only, the read is assigned to that gene. If the read's exons overlap exons of multiple annotated genes on the same strand, SpliceHunter tries to resolve ambiguity by picking the gene with largest overlap:

```
-u/--uniq <float>
```

If a read's exons overlap exons of multiple annotated genes on the same strand, SpliceHunter tries to resolve ambiguity by picking the gene with largest overlap, provided its overlap is at least <float> times larger than the second largest overlap with another gene. Default: 1.5.

If the read overlaps multiple annotated genes on different strands, SpliceHunter first tries to resolve ambiguity for each strand independently following the above strategy. If SpliceHunter successfully resolved ambiguity on both strands, it picks one strand based on thresholds adjusted by the following options:

```
-o/--ovsam <float>
```

If the overlap with the resolved gene g+ on the sense strand is at least <float> times larger than the largest overlap with a gene on the antisense strand, the read is assigned to gene g+. Default: 0.9.

```
-d/--ovdiff <float>
```

If a read could not be assigned to a gene on the sense strand, SpliceHunter assigns the read to the resolved gene on the antisense strand with largest overlap, provided this overlap is at least <float> times larger than the largest overlap with a gene on the sense strand. Default: 2.0.

If SpliceHunter managed to resolve gene ambiguity on the sense or antisense strand only, the overlap with the gene on that strand must again be larger than the largest overlap with a gene on the other strand by a factor determined by options `--ovsam` or `--ovdiff`, respectively. If a read does not overlap any annotated gene on either strand it will be used to infer novel transcription units.

3.3.4 Clustering Reads to Isoforms

After reads have been assigned to annotated genes or novel TUs, SpliceHunter clusters (transitively) compatible reads and merges them to putative isoforms. Two reads are compatible if they have been assigned to the same gene, if they align across or retain the exact same (potentially empty) set of introns, and if their start and end sites lie in a window of adjustable size. All compatible reads in the same cluster then form an isoform with start and end site corresponding to the most 5' start and most 3' end site among all reads in that cluster, respectively.

```
-t/-twin <int>
```

Snap start and end sites of a read to most 5' start site or most 3' end site within window of size <int> bases, respectively. Value −1 sets window size to infinity. Default: 50.

Reads with start or end site close to the annotated TSS or TES of the corresponding gene, respectively, form their own clusters:

```
-s/--snap <int>
```

Snap start and end sites of a read assigned to a gene g to the annotated TSS and TES of gene g if they lie within distance <int> bases. Set to −1 to turn off. Default: 50.

Similarly, novel TUs are inferred from clusters of reads that do not overlap any annotated gene and that all agree in their introns and have start and end sites close to each other (option `--twin`). Single exon reads form novel TUs by nonzero overlap alone. On request, SpliceHunter provides certificates for each predicted isoform:

```
-c/--cert
```

SpliceHunter provides certificates for each predicted isoform in file `certificates.txt`. A certificate lists, separately for each time point, all Iso-Seq read names (QNAME) from the input .bam files that are contained in the isoform's read cluster.

We provide a script for the visualization of certificates, *see* Subheading 3.4, **step 7**.

3.3.5 AS Events in Isoforms

Finally, the intron chain of each isoform is compared to the annotated exon–intron structure of the gene it has been assigned to detect alternative splicing events of the following type. Exon skippings and intron retentions refer to introns and exons in the novel isoform that fully contain at least one complete exon or intron of the reference transcript, respectively. Exon inclusions and introns in exons are the reverse events with the roles of the novel isoform and the reference transcript swapped. Alternative acceptors and donors appear exclusively in the novel isoform as the 3' and 5' ends of an intron, respectively. Novel exons do not overlap any exon of the reference transcript but are not spanned by any of its introns (*see* exon inclusions). Formal definitions of all AS events can be found in Kuang 2017 GR [5]. SpliceHunter writes novel TUs and all inferred isoforms along with their sequence of AS events to the console ("standard out"). Furthermore, SpliceHunter can provide read counts used in the analysis of pairwise dependencies of AS events as well as donor and acceptor sequences and the length of introns:

```
-j/--pwcount <pw_counts.txt>
```

SpliceHunter writes the four types of read counts for pairs of alternative splicing events into file `<pw_counts.txt>`. Default: off

```
-x/--hexamer <hexamer.txt>
```

SpliceHunter writes donor and acceptor hexamer sequences of all introns in detected isoforms into file `<hexamers.txt>`. Default: off

```
-i/--dimer <dimers.txt>
```

SpliceHunter writes donor and acceptor dimer sequences of all introns in detected isoforms into file `<dimers.txt>`. Default: off

```
-n/--retlength <retint_length.txt>
```

SpliceHunter writes the lengths of all retained introns into file `<retint_length.txt>`. Default: off

```
-z/--annoint <anno_introns.txt>
```

SpliceHunter outputs donor and acceptor hexamer sequences as well as the length of all annotated introns into file `<anno_introns.txt>`. Default: off

3.3.6 *Isoform Sequences*   For conservation analysis, SpliceHunter outputs the full RNA sequence of isoforms and TUs as well as their putative protein sequences to FASTA files:

```
-p/--protfile <protein_seq.fa>
```

SpliceHunter translates inferred isoforms of known genes and novel TUs and writes their sequences and longest ORFs, respectively, into FASTA file `<protein_seq.fa>`. Default: protseq.fa

```
-r/--rnafile <novel_rna_seq.fa>
```

SpliceHunter writes the RNA sequence of novel TUs into FASTA file `<novel_rna_seq.fa>`. Default: novel_rna.fa

```
-A/--asfile <as_rna_seq.fa>
```

SpliceHunter writes the RNA sequence of novel isoforms of known genes into FASTA file `<as_rna_seq.fa>`. Default: as_rna.fa

```
-y/--ncprotseq <reference_annotation.gtf>
```

SpliceHunter translates all genes in `<reference_annotation.gtf>` and writes their longest ORFs into FASTA file nc_protseq.fa. This option can be used to study hypothetical protein sequences of special transcript categories, like noncoding RNAs. Default: off

To run SpliceHunter on our sample data, extract archive `spombe_meiosis_rep1.tgz`, change to directory `spombe_-data`, and run SpliceHunter on the data from replicate 1:

```
tar -zxvf spombe_meiosis_rep1.tgz
cd spombe_data
SpliceHunter -g Spombe.ASM294v2.29.gtf -f allChr.fa -m ./rep1
-I isoforms.txt -c certificates.txt
```

This should create files `isoforms.txt`, `certificates.txt`, `protseq.fa`, `as_rna.fa`, `novel_rna.fa`, and `ambiguous.txt`, in the current directory.

3.4 Output Analysis

In this section, we describe several useful types of isoform analyses based on the output files of SpliceHunter. SpliceHunter writes results into tab-delimited files, which can be further processed and analyzed by various programming tools. Here, we provide an R script for users without extensive programming skills to facilitate the downstream analysis of inferred isoforms.

1. **Setting up R**: Open R and change the working directory to the folder which includes SpliceHunter's output files, the GTF annotation files, and the R source code.

2. **Load functions**: All functions are implemented in the FUNCTIONS section at the end of the script starting at line 78. Select all code defining the functions and execute it. Available

functions include `ASlandscape`, `ASperisoform`, `Isoview`, `Isodynamics`, and `ASassociation`, which we describe in more detail below.

3. **Load and preprocess data**: Replace the paths of example files with the paths to your SpliceHunter output files on line 2 and 13. Specify the number of time points (line 8) and replicates (line 9) accordingly and adjust the minimum required read count of an isoform to be considered in line 10. Execute the code from line 1 to line 52.

4. **AS landscape**: Execute line 55: `isoformlandsca-pe<-ASlandscape(isonew,mincount=1)`. Function `ASlandscape` takes two arguments, `isonew` and `mincount`. Data frame `isonew` is generated during the data preprocessing step and contains all isoforms and their splicing annotation required by `ASlandscape`. The `mincount` value can be specified by the user in line 10. Its default value is 1, that is, isoforms supported by at least 1 read are considered when determining the alternative splicing landscape. The function outputs a list object with two elements. The first element lists all detected AS events and the second element quantifies the occurrences of AS events by the number of supporting reads. Both elements are tables with rows representing different types of AS, and with one column for each time point. The last columns sum the number of AS events and their supporting reads over all time points, respectively. The AS landscape can be illustrated by a pie chart, which can be generated by executing line 58 (Fig. 2).

   Furthermore, we provide function `ASperisoform` to calculate the number of AS events per isoform. Execute line 61 to obtain the function's result as a table.

5. **Isoform structure and dynamics**: A common task in the analysis of alternative splicing is to explore the splicing pattern and the dynamics of a particular isoform or of a set of isoforms expressed by a gene of interest. We provide function `Isoview`

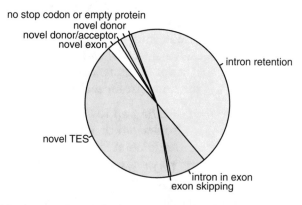

Fig. 2 AS landscape of example data generated by ASlandscape

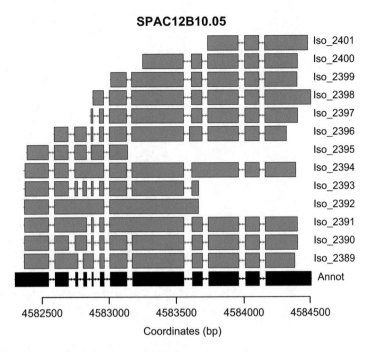

Fig. 3 Isoform structures of gene SPAC12B10.05 as generated by `Isoview`

to facilitate the visualization of one or multiple isoforms that belong to the same gene. Function `Isoview` expects an id assigned to an isoform by SpliceHunter, a vector of isoform ids, or a gene name as input and plots exon–intron structures of the isoforms given by their ids or all expressed isoforms of the given gene, respectively. Exons are denoted by rectangles that are connected by lines representing the introns. Arrows mark the direction of transcription. Annotated structures are colored in black and isoforms inferred by SpliceHunter are colored in blue. The associated id of each isoform is shown on the right side. Lines 64–66 in our R script provide examples for the different modes of usage of function `Isoview`. The execution of line 66 produces Fig. 3.

Function `Isodynamics` can be used to visualize the temporal patterns of isoforms across different time points or conditions. It takes as its first argument the IDs of one or multiple isoforms. The second argument `annot` specifies whether (`TRUE`) or not (`FALSE`) to plot the temporal pattern of the corresponding annotated isoform. By default `annot=FALSE`, i.e., the plot omits the annotated isoform. The execution of line 69 in our R script gives Fig. 4.

6. **Association analysis**: From long reads produced by PacBio sequencing, SpliceHunter infers isoforms long enough to span multiple AS events, allowing the study of their intramolecular association. We provide function `ASassociation` to

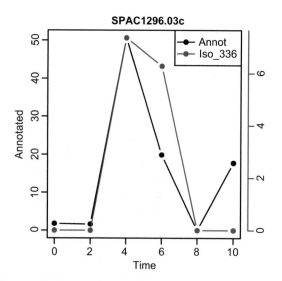

Fig. 4 The dynamics of the annotated isoform of gene SPAC1296.03c and isoform Iso_336 detected by SpliceHunter from the example data

quantify the association between pairs of AS events. For pairs of AS events that are each supported by 5–95% of all spanning reads, SpliceHunter outputs (option --pwcount) a vector of four elements, counting the numbers of reads supporting their coexistence, their coabsence, and their mutual exclusion, respectively. Function ASassociation returns a three-column table with rows corresponding to the tested AS pairs. The first column contains the P value from Fisher's exact test of independence of the two AS events. The second column gives the P values adjusted for the number of tested pairs via FDR. The third column quantifies the association by a score that is defined as the ratio of the number of reads supporting coexistence or coabsence to the total number of reads spanning both AS event. A high score close to 1 suggests coassociation of the events while a low score close to 0 indicates that they are mutually exclusive. In our example, we identified 153 pairs of coassociated introns with FDR < 0.05.

7. **Certificates**: SpliceHunter is able to provide certificates (option --cert) for its core functionality that can be used to visualize the dynamics of novel isoforms, in comparison to annotated gene structures, across time points or conditions. A certificate lists all Iso-Seq read names that are contained in the isoform's read cluster, split by time point or condition. Given the id of a novel TU or a novel isoform, script certifiate2-bam.sh uses the certificate to extract the corresponding alignments from the .bam file. It creates a separate .bam file for each time point or condition, sorts and indexes it, and prepares their color-coding in IGV.

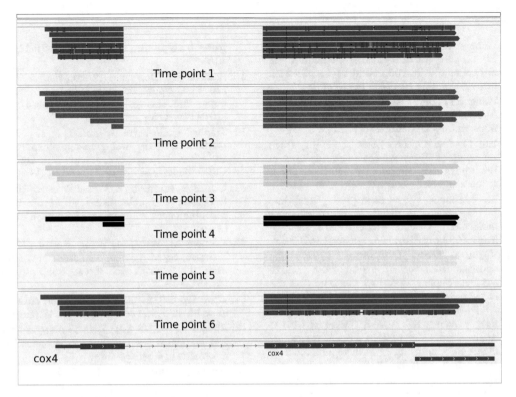

Fig. 5 IGV screenshot for the certificate of Iso_335

(a) Set variable `DIR` in file `certifiate2bam.sh` to the directory containing the input .bam files (used as argument `--dir`).

(b) Set variable `SAMPLE` to the list of samples and needs to match precisely the 8th column in the header of file `<isoform_file.txt>` if option `--iso` is used or "standard out" otherwise.

(c) Run `certifiate2bam.sh` and feed it with the certificate of the isoform of interest:

`grep -Ew '^Iso_335' certificates.txt | sh create_-cert.sh`. In this example, the certificate for isoform `Iso_335` is used to create 6 sorted .bam files `iso_[0--5].sorted.bam` and corresponding indexes.

(d) Load all .bam files into IGV to visualize the dynamics of the isoform of interest. Figure 5 shows an IGV screenshot for `Iso_335` in our sample data.

Acknowledgment

We thank Jef D. Boeke for critical reading of the manuscript.

References

1. Wang Z, Burge CB (2008) Splicing regulation: from a parts list of regulatory elements to an integrated splicing code. RNA 14(5):802–813. https://doi.org/10.1261/rna.876308

2. Wang ET, Sandberg R, Luo S et al (2008) Alternative isoform regulation in human tissue transcriptomes. Nature 456(7221):470–476

3. Pan Q, Shai O, Lee LJ et al (2008) Deep surveying of alternative splicing complexity in the human transcriptome by high-throughput sequencing. Nat Genet 40(12):1413–1415

4. Eid J, Fehr A, Gray J et al (2009) Real-time DNA sequencing from single polymerase molecules. Science 323(5910):133–138. https://doi.org/10.1126/science.1162986

5. Kuang Z, Boeke JD, Canzar S (2017) The dynamic landscape of fission yeast meiosis alternative-splice isoforms. Genome Res 27 (1):145–156. https://doi.org/10.1101/gr.208041.116

6. Katz Y, Wang ET, Airoldi EM et al (2010) Analysis and design of RNA sequencing experiments for identifying isoform regulation. Nat Methods 7(12):1009–1015

7. Shen S, Park JW, Huang J et al (2012) MATS: a Bayesian framework for flexible detection of differential alternative splicing from RNA-Seq data. Nucleic Acids Res 40(8):e61. https://doi.org/10.1093/nar/gkr1291

8. Brooks AN, Yang L, Duff MO et al (2011) Conservation of an RNA regulatory map between drosophila and mammals. Genome Res 21(2):193–202. https://doi.org/10.1101/gr.108662.110

9. Wang Q, Rio D (2017) The junction usage model (JUM): a method for comprehensive annotation-free differential analysis of tissue-specific global alternative pre-mRNA splicing patterns. bioRxiv. https://doi.org/10.1101/116863

10. Branton D, Deamer DW, Marziali A et al (2008) The potential and challenges of nanopore sequencing. Nat Biotechnol 26 (10):1146–1153

11. Trapnell C, Roberts A, Goff L et al (2012) Differential gene and transcript expression analysis of RNA-seq experiments with TopHat and cufflinks. Nat Protoc 7(3):562–578

12. Canzar S, Andreotti S, Weese D et al (2016) CIDANE: comprehensive isoform discovery and abundance estimation. Genome Biol 17 (1):16

13. Källberg M, Wang H, Wang S et al (2012) Template-based protein structure modeling using the RaptorX web server. Nat Protoc 7 (8):1511–1522

14. Team RC (2015). R: a language and environment for statistical computing. Vienna, Austria

15. Rhoads A, Au KF (2015) PacBio sequencing and its applications. Genomics Proteomics Bioinformatics 13(5):278–289

16. Wu TD, Watanabe CK (2005) GMAP: a genomic mapping and alignment program for mRNA and EST sequences. Bioinformatics 21 (9):1859–1875. bti310 [pii]

17. Robinson JT, Thorvaldsdóttir H, Winckler W et al (2011) Integrative genomics viewer. Nat Biotechnol 29(1):24–26

18. Canzar S (2017) Example data used in this tutorial. https://syncandshare.lrz.de/dl/fiLzMSDfnrhLZ8MoiirvqAza/spombe_meiosis_rep1.tgz

19. Camacho C, Coulouris G, Avagyan V et al (2009) BLAST: architecture and applications. BMC Bioinformatics 10(1):421

Chapter 6

RNA-Seq-Based Transcript Structure Analysis with TrBorderExt

Yejun Wang, Ming-an Sun, and Aaron P. White

Abstract

RNA-Seq has become a routine strategy for genome-wide gene expression comparisons in bacteria. Despite lower resolution in transcript border parsing compared with dRNA-Seq, TSS-EMOTE, Cappable-seq, Term-seq, and others, directional RNA-Seq still illustrates its advantages: low cost, quantification and transcript border analysis with a medium resolution (± 10–20 nt). To facilitate mining of directional RNA-Seq datasets especially with respect to transcript structure analysis, we developed a tool, TrBorderExt, which can parse transcript start sites and termination sites accurately in bacteria. A detailed protocol is described in this chapter for how to use the software package step by step to identify bacterial transcript borders from raw RNA-Seq data. The package was developed with Perl and R programming languages, and is accessible freely through the website: http://www.szu-bioinf.org/TrBorderExt.

Key words Directional RNA-Seq, Transcript unit, Operon, Transcript border, Transcript start site, Transcript termination site

1 Introduction

Dramatic advances in the resolving power of DNA sequencing technology and decreasing costs have revolutionized bacterial transcriptome studies. RNA-Seq can generate large-scale gene expression data at single-nucleotide resolution that allow both quantitative expression comparisons and qualitative analysis on biological features in a strand specific manner such as transcript border definition and sRNA identification [1, 2]. At present, however, RNA-Seq experiments with bacteria are mostly used for a quantitative objective in a majority of laboratories [3–5].

Genes are condensed in bacterial genomes, and the structure of transcripts is not as complex as in eukaryotic organisms. Consequently, once a bacterial genome is sequenced, gene models can be computationally annotated with high accuracy. However, similar to humans or other eukaryotes, bacterial transcriptomes have been observed to have high dynamics, not merely in expression level

Yejun Wang and Ming-an Sun (eds.), *Transcriptome Data Analysis: Methods and Protocols*, Methods in Molecular Biology, vol. 1751, https://doi.org/10.1007/978-1-4939-7710-9_6, © Springer Science+Business Media, LLC 2018

but also in the structure of transcripts [6–8]. Overlaps between nontranslated regions and coding fragments of adjacent genes are frequently observed in bacteria, causing gene frame-based expression quantification and comparisons to be inaccurate [9]. Therefore, transcript border identification and transcription unit-based quantification appeared more appropriate. Bacterial genomes are organized in operons, so the core of transcriptional structure analysis is to annotate the operon architecture. In practice, an operon is defined by the transcript start site (TSS) and the transcript termination site (TTS), and therefore identification of the TSSs and TTSs becomes the focus of RNA-Seq-based operon architecture analysis.

Predominant RNA-Seq experiments have many advantages in quantitative studies, but meanwhile have inherent drawbacks for transcript border analysis [10]. New technologies, e.g., differential RNA-Seq (dRNA-Seq), TSS-EMOTE, Cappable-seq and Term-seq, have facilitated more accurate location of the TSSs and TTSs [11–14]. The ideal design for bacterial transcriptome research would include both dRNA-Seq/TSS-EMOTE/Cappable-seq, Term-seq and typical directional RNA-Seq experiments, following the analytic pipeline shown in Fig. 1. In an absolute majority of laboratories, however, only directional (i.e., strand-specific) RNA--Seq experiments are performed. Therefore, a tool is desired to perform both qualitative annotation and quantitative analysis of bacterial transcriptomes based only on directional RNA-Seq data. Previously, we developed a software package, TrBorderExt, which was designed specifically for transcript border identification based on directional RNA-Seq data [10]. TrBorderExt could not locate the TSSs as accurately as dRNA-Seq-based analysis because of the inherent limits of RNA-Seq, and yet the structure for most operons could be resolved within ~10–20 nucleotides [10]. We have illustrated a typical design for bacterial transcriptome studies and listed some analytic methods (Fig. 1; [15–18]). For these methods, readers are referred to the references listed and to other chapters in the book that address specific objectives of bacterial transcriptome analysis. Due to the length limit of this chapter, below we have illustrated how to use TrBorderExt exclusively to analyze transcript borders.

2   Materials

2.1   RNA-Seq Data Sets

The RNA-Seq data from a *Salmonella* transcriptome study (no. SRP056892) were used for testing the protocol (https://www.ncbi.nlm.nih.gov/sra). The study contained eight datasets SRX976427, SRX976344, SRX976343, SRX976341, SRX976337, SRX976336, SRX976335, and SRX974437, each representing different time point or biological phenotypes. The

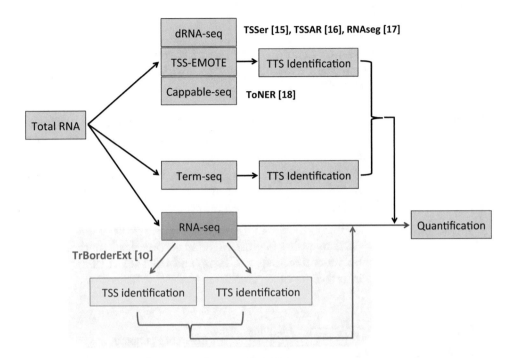

Fig. 1 Design and analysis of bacterial transcriptome. An ideal design was shown in grey box, with dRNA-Seq/ TSS-EMOTE/Cappable-seq and Term-seq in the first place for TSS and TTS identification respectively, followed by directional RNA-Seq and transcript unit quantification. The TSSer, TSSAR, RNAseg, and ToNER are software tools that automatically analyze TSSs from the TSS-enriched RNA-Seq data [15–18]. There are no tools currently available for automatically analyzing Term-seq data. In most typical RNA-Seq experiments, only directional RNA-Seq data are available (blue box), and TrBorderExt can be used to extract TSSs and TTSs (in red). The transcript borders identified with TrBorderExt could be used to update the transcript structure and make more accurate quantification of the genes

reads were directional and paired-end, generated from an Illumina HiSeq 2000 platform.

2.2 Reference Genome and Annotation

The genome sequence of *Salmonella typhimurium* strain 14028S and the annotation file were downloaded from NCBI GenBank database (Accession: NC_016856.1).

2.3 Software Tools

Geneious was installed for implementing read-genome mapping and preparation of preprocessed files (http://www.geneious.com/). TrBorderExt package (for Windows or Linux/Mac) could be downloaded from the website: http://www.szu-bioinf.org/ TrBorderExt. Decompress the package directly. Installation of Perl 5.0 or a later version is a prerequisite for running TrBorderExt (https://www.perl.org/). R is an optional prerequisite if the user wishes to determine the statistically reliable transcript units. Download R from http://www.r-project.org and install it according to the documents.

3   Methods

As shown in Fig. 2, analysis of bacterial transcript borders from directional RNA-Seq data with TrBorderExt is quite straightforward.

3.1   Preprocessing of RNA-Seq Data

1. Open Geneious, an interfaced sequence analysis software tool. Copy the directional RNA-Seq data and reference bacterial genome GenBank file into Geneious (*see* **Note 1**).

2. Select an RNA-Seq data file to be analyzed. In the main interface of Geneious, select "Tools" → "Align/Assemble" → "Map to reference …", and then indicate the reference file. Set the parameters and then run read-genome mapping (*see* **Note 2**).

3. After mapping is finished, a file automatically named *Contig* will be generated. Select *Contig*, and then select "File" in the main interface of Geneious → "Export" → "Select

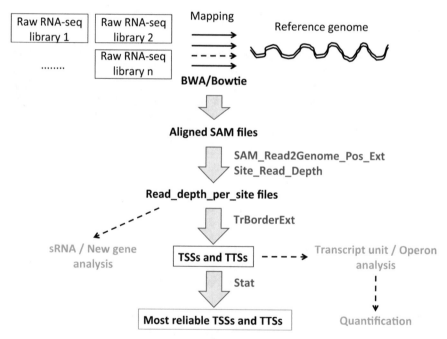

Fig. 2 Pipeline of transcript border analysis with TrBorderExt. RNA-Seq libraries need to be mapped to reference genomes with alignment tools such as *BWA*, *Bowtie* or DNA analysis software programs like Geneious (Biomatters Inc.), as described here. The aligned files in SAM format are further analyzed with *SAM_Read2Genome_Pos_Ext* and *Site_Read_Depth* scripts in the TrBorderExt package to parse the read depth per site. The read depth (per site) files can be used for transcript border parsing with TrBorderExt or for analysis of sRNAs or new genes (shown in grey type). The TSSs and TTSs identified with TrBorderExt can be used directly for transcript unit or operon analysis and subsequent transcript unit quantification. To extract the more statistically reliable TSSs and TTSs from *TrBorderExt* results, *Stat* can be further applied. The tools or modules available in TrBorderExt are highlighted in red

Documents..." → "SAM sequence alignment/map files (*.sam)". Designate the file to be generated and indicate the directory where the file will be stored.

4. Repeat **steps 2** and **3** for each RNA-Seq data file to be analyzed.

3.2 Analysis of Read Depth per Site

1. Download the TrBorderExt software package. When fully decompressed, this package contains the following subdirectories—"bin", "stat", "Accessory_scripts", and "Example", and the files—'DOCUMENT.txt', "TrBorderExt.pl", and "stat.pl".

2. Create a new folder (for example, in Linux, "/home/rnaseq/"). Transfer the SAM files generated in Subheading 3.1 into the folder, along with the scripts "*SAM_Read2Genome_Pos_Ext_P.pl*", "*SAM_Read2Genome_Pos_Ext_S.pl*", and "*Site_Read_Depth.pl*" found in subdirectory "Accessory_scripts" of the TrBorderExt package. Copy the decompressed directory "TrBorderExt_linux" (or "TrBorderExt_win") completely into the working folder.

3. Run "*SAM_Read2Genome_Pos_Ext*" to parse the genomic coordinates of RNA-Seq reads. For Linux and Illumina paired-end reads, running the following commands:

```
$ cd /home/rnseq/
$ perl SAM_Read2Genome_Pos_Ext_P.pl <MAPPING_SAM_FILE>
>READ_COORD_FILE
```

The MAPPING_SAM_FILEs were the aligned files generated in Subheading 3.1. For single-end reads, use "*SAM_Read2Genome_Pos_Ext_S.pl*" to replace the script "*SAM_Read2Genome_Pos_Ext_P.pl*". Similar scripts and procedure were used in the DOS interface of Windows operation system.

4. Run "*Site_Read_Depth.pl*" to calculate the depth of each genomic position covered by RNA-Seq reads.

```
$ perl Site_Read_Depth.pl < READ_COORD_FILE> REF_SIZE
>SITE_READ_DEPTH_FILE
```

READ_COORD_FILE was generated in Subheading 3.2, **step 2**, and REF_SIZE is the length of reference genome with the resolution of 1 nucleotide. The generated SITE_READ_DEPTH_FILE will be used for further transcript border analysis. The file format is shown in Fig. 3.

5. Move SITE_READ_DEPTH_FILE into the TrBorderExt package folder (e.g.,"/home/rnaseq/TrBorderExt_linux/").

6. Repeat **steps 2–4** for each RNA-Seq library.

3.3 Parsing the Borders of Transcript Units

1. Prepare gene tab file for which the format is shown in Fig. 3. The script 'GB.parse.pl' in the subdirectory "Accessory_scripts" of the TrBorderExt package could help prepare the gene tab file

Format of SITE_READ_DEPTH_FILE

Coordinate	Forward_Coverage	Reverse_Coverage
1	10	0
2	12	0
3	11	0
...	...	...
GENOME_SIZE	XXX	XXX

Format of GENE_TAB_FILE

thrL	190-255	+
thrA	337-2799	+
thrB	2801-3730	+
thrC	3734-5020	+
yaaA	5114-5887	-
yaaJ	5966-7396	-
talB	7665-8618	+
mogA	8729-9319	+
yaaH	9376-9942	-
htgA	10092-10805	-
yaaI	10841-11245	-
STM14_0012	11257-11424	+
...	...	...

Fig. 3 The format of "site_read_depth" and "gene_tab" files used as part of the TrBorderExt pipeline. SITE_READ_DEPTH_FILE contains three columns: the genome coordinate (1); Forward_coverage (2) and Reverse_coverage (3) refer to the read depth in the sense or antisense genomic strands, respectively, at each corresponding genomic position. GENE_TAB_FILE also contains three columns: (1) gene name; (2) the start and ending positions of the gene CDS; and (3) the genomic strand where the gene is located (sense (+), antisense (−))

(*see* **Note 3**). Move the GENE_TAB_FILE into the TrBorderExt package folder (e.g., "/home/rnaseq/TrBorderExt_linux/").

2. One-step transcript border parsing for each library.

```
$ cd  /home/rnseq/TrBorderExt_linux/
$ perl   TrBorderExt.pl   <SITE_READ_DEPTH_FILE>
<GENE_TAB_FILE>  REF_SIZE
CUSTOMIZED_LIBRARY_NAME
```

CUSTOMIZED_LIBRARY_NAME is a simple identifier indicated for each library. Two files will be generated eventually, with "CUSTOMIZED_LIBRARY_NAME.all.TSS.txt" representing all the transcript start sites and "CUSTOMIZED_LIBRARY_-NAME.all.TSS.txt" representing all the transcript termination sites. The format of generated files is shown in Fig. 4. Six different types of TSS or TTS were identified and described previously [10], based on the TSS/TTS read coverage and the relative read abundance (signal-to-noise ratio) between TSS/TTS and adjacent genomic sites. A diagram was also presented to explain the TSS/TTS types (Fig. 5).

Gene	Str	Type	TSS/TTS	B_Cov	Cov	CDS_st	Location
thrL	+	1	148	0	4	190	Intergenic
talB	+	1	8191	0	8	8238	Intergenic
fkpB	+	2	25756	0	1	25826	Intergenic
dapB	+	2	28290	0	1	28374	Intergenic
carA	+	2	29550	0	1	29651	Intergenic
cra	+	1	87969	0	8	88028	Intergenic
mraZ	+	1	89597	0	2	89634	Intergenic
ampD	+	2	118701	0	1	118733	Intergenic
pdhR	+	1	122034	0	6	122092	Intergenic
aceE	+	1	122969	0	25	123017	Intergenic
lpd	+	2	127616	0	1	127912	Intergenic
...	...	...	...	...	...	...	...

Fig. 4 The format of TSS or TTS identification files. Str, Strand; Type, TSS/TTS category (1–6) based on the site coverage and signal-to-noise ratio between coverage of TSS/TTS and adjacent sites; TSS/TTS, the corresponding genomic coordinates; B_Cov and Cov, border coverage and TSS/TTS coverage respectively; CDS_st, the start site of corresponding gene CDS; Location, relative location of the TSS/TTS to corresponding gene (Intergenic or Ingenic)

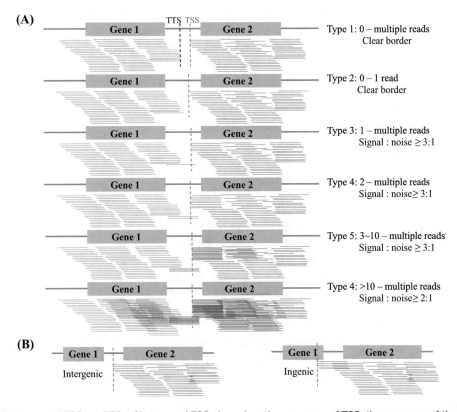

Fig. 5 The types of TSSs or TTSs. Six types of TSSs based on the coverage of TSS, the coverage of the border and the ratio were shown in (**a**). For each type, the first number listed refers to the number of reads covering the genomic position 1-nt before the TSS of Gene 2 (border) and the second number refers to the number of reads mapped to the TSS of Gene 2 transcript. The signal-to-noise ratio refers to the second number divided by the first number. For TTSs, there were the same six types. (**b**) The TSSs/TTSs were also classified as Intergenic or Ingenic, depending on the TSS/TTS location (between two known gene frames, or within a known gene frame)

In the one-step protocol, all the parameters were set as default, e.g., no less than 75% length of a transcript being covered by at least 1 read. However, Some researchers may wish to examine flexible parameters. Therefore, an alternative protocol was also provided to perform stepwise transcript border analysis, and the users can modify the parameters in command lines.

3. Stepwise transcript border parsing for each library (**Alternative**, *see* **Note 4**).

```
$ cd   /home/rnseq/TrBorderExt_linux/
$ perl ./bin/geneUTR_tab.pl <GENE_TAB_FILE> REF_SIZE >utr.txt
$ perl ./bin/UTRlength.filter.pl utr.txt 5 >utr_5.txt
$ perl ./bin/UTRlength.filter.pl utr.txt 500 >utr_all.txt
$ perl ./bin/geneCoverageStat.pl <SITE_READ_DEPTH_FILE>
  <GENE_TAB_FILE> >sample.gene.coverage.txt
$ perl ./bin/geneCoverageFilter.pl sample.gene.coverage.txt 3
0.75 >sample.3_75.filter.tab.txt
$ perl ./bin/geneUTR_Cover.JointFilter.pl sample.3_75.filter.
tab.txt
  utr_5.txt >sample.3_75_L5.tab.txt
$ perl ./bin/geneUTR_Cover.JointFilter.pl sample.3_75.filter.
tab.txt
  utr_all.txt >sample.3_75_L_All.tab.txt
$ perl ./bin/geneStructureRetrieve.pl <SITE_READ_DEPTH_FILE>
sample.3_75_L5.tab.txt
  sample.3_75_L5
$ perl ./bin/geneStructureRetrieve2.pl <SITE_READ_DEPTH_FILE>
sample.3_75_L_All.tab.txt
  100 sample.3_75_L-100
$ perl ./bin/mergeTranscriptStructure.pl  sample.3_75_L5.TSS.
txt sample.3_75_L-100.TSS.txt
utr.txt >sample.all.TSS.txt
$ perl ./bin/mergeTranscriptStructure.pl  sample.3_75_L5.TTS.
txt sample.3_75_L-100.TTS.txt
  utr.txt >sample.all.TTS.txt
$ rm utr*
$ rm sample.3_75*
$ rm sample.gene.coverage.txt
$ mv sample.all.TSS.txt CUSTOMIZED_LIBRARY_NAME.all.TSS.txt
$ mv sample.all.TTS.txt CUSTOMIZED_LIBRARY_NAME.all.TTS.txt
```

3.4 Statistical Analysis of the Accuracy of Transcript Borders Identified Using TrBorderExt

This step is optional (*see* **Note 5**), but recommended to determine the degree of confidence for specific TSS or TTS. In our opinion, if a researcher has sequenced multiple libraries, then statistical analysis should be performed. It should be noted, however, that although this will increase the precision, it does result in a small loss of sensitivity.

1. Put all the transcript border files ("CUSTOMIZED_SAM-PLE_NAME.all.TSS.txt" and "CUSTOMIZED_SAMPLE_-NAME.all.TTS.txt") in current directory.

2. Use "stat.pl" to do the statistical analysis. Two options are provided for statistical testing, "Read" or "Sample" (or both). It is suggested to perform "Read"-based statistical test.

```
$ cd  /home/rnseq/TrBorderExt_linux/
$ perl  stat.pl  TEST_TYPE
```

TEST_TYPE should be "Read", "Sample", or "Both", for read-based, sample-based, or both types of statistical test. At least four files will be generated: (1) "All_sample.combined_TSS.txt", (2) "All_sample.combined_TTS.txt", (3) "TSS.read_test.txt" (or "TSS.sample_test.txt"), and (4) "TTS.read_test.txt" (or "TTS.sample_test.txt").

4   Notes

1. In this protocol, BWA integrated in Geneious was used for RNA-Seq mapping. In practice, however, researchers can directly use free, publically available short-read mapping tools such as *BWA* or *Bowtie*.

2. The mapping parameters can be adjusted based on the quality of the raw reads, the read length, the overall sequencing depth and the genome complexity. In the protocol outlined, full length reads were rejected if there were >5% mismatches or if repeats were present, i.e., one read mapped to two genome regions meanwhile.

3. The Gene_tab file should be parsed in advance, with a format indicated in Fig. 3. A script "GB.parse.pl" was also developed and stored in the subdirectory "Accessory_scripts" of the TrBorderExt package, which could help prepare the gene tab file. Please note that the script only parses protein-encoding genes and ncRNAs. Before using "GB.parse.pl", the GenBank file (GB_FILE) of corresponding reference genome should be downloaded from NCBI Genome database or elsewhere and stored in current directory. The usage was shown below:

```
USAGE: perl GB.parse.pl <GB_FILE>
Example: $ perl GB.parse.pl NC_000913.gb >K-12.gene.tab.txt
```

4. The transcript borders could be parsed with TrBorderExt by one step. However, TrBorderExt is a pipeline with sequential sub-steps, for each of which the script was stored in the subdirectory "bin". The purpose for each substep was shown in the annotation lines of the corresponding scripts. Users could also modify the parameters in individual scripts for specific bacterial species or research objectives.

5. Binomial tests were used for reliability evaluation of the TSSs and TTSs. However, as described in reference [10] and elsewhere, the inherent deficiencies of directional RNA-Seq techniques, particularly without $5'/3'$-end protection or enrichment, determined that the resolution of TSS/TTS identification can only be within ~10–20 nucleotides. Statistical tests will not improve the resolution; however, they will reduce the uncertainty caused by random sampling bias.

Acknowledgment

This work was supported by a Natural Science Funding of Shenzhen (JCYJ201607115221141) and a Shenzhen Peacock Plan fund (827-000116) to YW. The funders had no role in study design, data collection and analysis, decision to publish, or preparation of the manuscript.

References

1. Creecy JP, Conway T (2015) Quantitative bacterial transcriptomics with RNA-Seq. Curr Opin Microbiol 23:133–140

2. Kröger C, Dillon SC, Cameron ADS, Papenfort K, Sivasankaran SK, Hokamp K, Chao Y, Sittka A, Hébrard M, Händler K et al (2012) The transcriptional landscape and small RNAs of salmonella enterica serovar Typhimurium. Proc Natl Acad Sci 109: E1277–E1286

3. Wright MS, Jacobs MR, Bonomo RA, Adams MD (2017) Transcriptome remodeling of acinetobacter baumannii during infection and treatment. MBio 8(2):e02193–e02116

4. Zhao F, Wang Y, An H, Hao Y, Hu X, Liao X (2016) New insights into the formation of viable but nonculturable Escherichia coli O157: H7 induced by high-pressure CO_2. MBio 7(4): e00961–e00916

5. MacKenzie KD, Wang Y, Shivak DJ, Wong CS, Hoffman LJL, Lam S, Kröger C, Cameron ADS, Townsend HGG, Köster W (2015) Bistable expression of CsgD in salmonella enterica serovar Typhimurium connects virulence to persistence. Infect Immun 83:2312–2326

6. McGrath PT, Lee H, Zhang L, Iniesta AA, Hottes AK, Tan MH, Hillson NJ, Hu P, Shapiro L, McAdams HH (2007) High-throughput identification of transcription start sites, conserved promoter motifs and predicted regulons. Nat Biotechnol 25 (5):584–592

7. Cho BK, Zengler K, Qiu Y, Park YS, Knight EM, Barrett CL, Gao Y, Palsson BØ (2009) The transcription unit architecture of the Escherichia coli genome. Nat Biotechnol 27 (11):1043–1049

8. Mitschke J, Vioque A, Haas F, Hess WR, Muro-Pastor AM (2011) Dynamics of transcriptional start site selection during nitrogen stress-induced cell differentiation in anabaena sp. PCC7120. Proc Natl Acad Sci U S A 108 (50):20130–20135

9. Colgan AM, Cameron AD, Kröger C (2017) If it transcribes, we can sequence it: mining the complexities of host-pathogen-environment

interactions using RNA-Seq. Curr Opin Microbiol 36:37–46

10. Wang Y, MacKenzie KD, White AP (2015) An empirical strategy to detect bacterial transcript structure from directional RNA-Seq transcriptome data. BMC Genomics 16:359

11. Sharma CM, Hoffmann S, Darfeuille F, Reignier J, Findeiss S, Sittka A, Chabas S, Reiche K, Hackermüller J, Reinhardt R, Stadler PF, Vogel J (2010) The primary transcriptome of the major human pathogen helicobacter pylori. Nature 464(7286):250–255

12. Prados J, Linder P, Redder P (2016) TSS-EMOTE, a refined protocol for a more complete and less biased global mapping of transcription start sites in bacterial pathogens. BMC Genomics 17:849

13. Ettwiller L, Buswell J, Yigit E, Schildkraut I (2016) A novel enrichment strategy reveals unprecedented number of novel transcription start sites at single base resolution in a model prokaryote and the gut microbiome. BMC Genomics 17:199

14. Dar D, Shamir M, Mellin JR, Koutero M, Stern-Ginossar N, Cossart P, Sorek R (2016) Term-seq reveals abundant ribo-regulation of antibiotics resistance in bacteria. Science 352 (6282):aad9822

15. Jorjani H, Zavolan M (2014) TSSer: an automated method to identify transcription start sites in prokaryotic genomes from differential RNA sequencing data. Bioinformatics 30 (7):971–974

16. Amman F, Wolfinger MT, Lorenz R, Hofacker IL, Stadler PF, Findeiß S (2014) TSSAR: TSS annotation regime for dRNA-Seq data. BMC Bioinformatics 15:89

17. Bischler T, Kopf M, Voß B (2014) Transcript mapping based on dRNA-Seq data. BMC Bioinformatics 15:122

18. Promworn Y, Kaewprommal P, Shaw PJ, Intarapanich A, Tongsima S, Piriyapongsa J (2017) ToNER: a tool for identifying nucleotide enrichment signals in feature-enriched RNA-Seq data. PLoS One 12(5):e0178483

## Chapter 7

Analysis of RNA Editing Sites from RNA-Seq Data Using GIREMI

Qing Zhang

Abstract

RNA editing is a posttranscriptional modification process that alters the sequence of RNA molecules. RNA editing is related to many human diseases. However, the identification of RNA editing sites typically requires matched genomic sequence or multiple related expression data sets. Here we describe the GIREMI tool (genome-independent identification of RNA editing by mutual information; https://github.com/zhqingit/giremi) that is designed to accurately and sensitively predict adenosine-to-inosine editing from a single RNA-Seq data set.

Key words RNA editing, RNA-Seq, Posttranscriptional modification

1 Introduction

RNA editing is a posttranscriptional modification process that alters the sequence of RNA molecules. When it occurs in the untranslated regions (UTRs) or exons, RNA editing modulates the RNA stability and the translation process [1]. The mice with the knockout of two RNA-editing enzyme-encoding genes, *Adar1* and *Adar2*, are embryonically and postnatally lethal, respectively [2, 3]. The RNA-editing deficiencies have been observed in epilepsy, amyotrophic lateral sclerosis (ALS), Aicardi–Goutieres syndrome (AGS), schizophrenia, suicidal depression, and other neurodegenerative diseases [4–6]. In addition, recent studies indicate that RNA editing process or site-specific editing is related to various cancers [7–10] and associated with patient survival [9].

Computational tools have been developed recently to detect RNA editing sites [11]. However, all of them require the matched genome sequence data in order to discriminate RNA editing sites (RNAE) from genomic single nucleotide polymorphisms (SNPs) [11]. Because of the nonuniformity in sequencing coverage or other issues, some SNPs still fail to be identified. In view of the different conservation levels of the RNA editing sites and SNPs, a

Yejun Wang and Ming-an Sun (eds.), *Transcriptome Data Analysis: Methods and Protocols*, Methods in Molecular Biology, vol. 1751, https://doi.org/10.1007/978-1-4939-7710-9_7, © Springer Science+Business Media, LLC 2018

new method was proposed to use multiple RNA-Seq data sets alone to find the RNA editing sites; however, it still precludes analysis of single data sets and may miss unique changes [12]. We devised a tool GIREMI (genome-independent identification of RNA editing by mutual information) that can separate the RNA editing sites from genomic variations (e.g., SNPs) based on single RNA-Seq datasets [13].

In this chapter, I provide a step-by-step protocol on how to use GIREMI to identify RNA editing sites from RNA-Seq data.

2 Materials

2.1 RNA-Seq Datasets and Reference Genome Sequences

The testing RNA-Seq dataset used for this protocol was accessible through the link: https://github.com/zhqingit/giremi. Download the compressed file ("test.fastq.gz").

The human reference genome sequences (GRCh37/hg19) were downloaded from UCSC: http://hgdownload.cse.ucsc.edu/goldenPath/hg19/.

2.2 Tools

1. Read mapping tool, BWA: http://bio-bwa.sourceforge.net/. Install and configure the tool according to the documents.

2. SAMtools: http://samtools.sourceforge.net/. Install and configure the tools according to the documents.

3. GIREMI could be downloaded through the link: https://github.com/zhqingit/giremi. The package is developed with R, Perl, Python, and C programming languages. There is a manual in the website that could be followed to install and configure GIREMI correctly.

2.3 System Requirements

BWA, SAMtools, and GIREMI all support Linux (Ubuntu, Red Hat, SUSE, and others) system. At least 8 GB of memory is required for GIREMI to process typical human datasets.

3 Methods

GERIME combines a mutual information (MI) based inference method with a generalized linear model (GLM) to predict the RNA editing sites. Taking the advantage of the high throughput sequencing technology, we can collect a set of SNV pairs located on the same reads ($> = 5$ reads). The pairs with different composition show variable behaviors. As shown in Fig. 1a, SNP/SNP pairs can pass the haplotype information on the reads. From the statistic viewpoint, the two sites are dependent. In contrast, RNA editing occurs post-transcriptionally and the mRNAs are randomly chosen to be edited, so the SNP/RNAE or RNAE/RNAE sites are

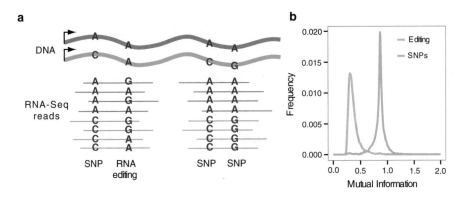

Fig. 1 The GIREMI method. (**a**) The allelic combinations of two SNPs in the same RNA-Seq reads are the same as their DNA haplotypes, whereas a SNP and an RNA editing site (or a pair of RNA editing sites) exhibit variable allelic linkage. (**b**) Distributions of mutual information associated with SNPs and RNA editing sites, estimated using GM12878 RNA-Seq data (ENCODE, cytosolic, poly(A) +) and its associated genome sequencing data. (Adapted from Figure 1 in Zhang et al. [13])

independent (Fig. 1a). The mutual information (MI) is a popular method to measure the dependence between two variables. The MI of different SNV pairs inferred by the RNA-Seq reads (Fig. 1b) shows totally different distributions. Based on the above evidences, we devise a method to identify the RNA editing sites using the RNA-Seq data alone (Fig. 2).

We firstly extract the known SNPs from the single nucleotide variants (SNVs) inferred from the RNA-Seq data based on the public databases. Then we build the MI distribution of these known SNP pairs. Any SNV whose MI value is out of this distribution is considered as RNAE. For some SNV sites, we cannot calculate their MI values because they are not covered by enough reads holding other SNV sites. So we apply a generalized linear models (GLM) trained by the known SNPs and MI-inferred RNAE to extend the predictive power of GIREMI (Fig. 2). Because the sequencing or PCR errors occur randomly on the reads, their MI values will be similar to that of the RNAE. Therefore, it is very important to remove the sequencing or PCR errors before using GIREMI.

3.1 Mapping of RNA-Seq Reads

RNA-Seq reads are mapped to human genome sequences or transcriptome using bowtie [14], bwa [15], blat [16], or other alignment tools.

```
CMD:    bwa aln hg19.fa test.fastq.gz > test.sai
        bwa samse hg19.fa test.sai test.fq > test.sam
```

Parameters can be specified based on the pair-end or single-end sequencing and the length of the reads. The mapping results are exported into a file with SAM format.

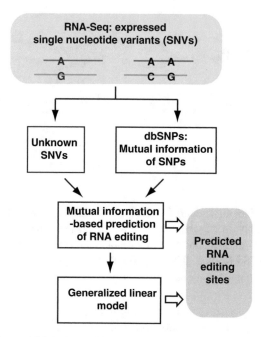

Fig. 2 Flowchart of GIREMI. GIREMI is designed to identify the RNA editing sites based on prealigned file and the known SNPs list. There are many methods to generate the alignment result (bam/sam file) from the raw RNA-Seq reads. These methods are very straightforward, and the user only needs run the commands. Below a test sample was used to illustrate the whole pipeline (Materials). (Adapted from Figure S1b in Zhang et al. [13])

3.2 Preprocessing to Identify and Filter Mismatches in RNA-Seq Reads

1. Remove the duplicates

The step can be done with GATK [17–19], SAMtools [20], or any other tool with similar applications. Here, SAMtools is used and shown as an example. First, the mapping result file (SAM format) generated from the Subheading 3.1 is transformed to BAM format and sorted, followed by removing the duplicates with the "rmdup" module of SAMtools.

```
CMD:    samtools view –Sb test.sam > test.bam
        samtools sort test.bam > test_sorted.bam
        samtools rmdup –S test_sorted.bam > test_dup.bam
```

2. Call SNVs

The SNVs are called from the duplicate-free BAM file obtained from last step. Sequencing and other errors are removed. GATK [17–19], SAMtools [20], or other tools can be applied. Here, we also use SAMtools as an example. Users can refer to the documents along with these tools to set the parameters.

```
CMD:    samtools mpileup –uf hg19.fa test_dup.bam | bcftools
        call –c –v | bcftools filter –i'DP>=5' > test.vcf
```

The SNVs are recorded in the resulting VCF file, which will be further parsed for the RNA editing sites with GIREMI.

3.3   Run GIREMI

1. Generate the list of SNVs with marked known SNPs

Download the human gene information ("ref_gene.txt") from UCSC table browser:

https://genome.ucsc.edu/cgi-bin/hgTables

Choose "Genes and Gene Predictions" for group and "all fields from selected tables" for output format.

Variations are annotated with snpEff, which can be downloaded from: http://snpeff.sourceforge.net/download.html. Make sure that snpEff use the same gene name as that in the ref_gene.txt. Use a custom script "mark_snp.py" downloaded from github website of GIREMI to generate the input file of GIREMEI curating the list of SNVs with marked known SNPs.

```
CMD:  java -Xmx4g -jar snpEff.jar hg19 test.vcf > test_ano.vcf
      mark_snp.py -s test.vcf -i test_ano.vcf -g ref_gene.txt >
      test.txt
```

2. Generate the RNA editing list

```
CMD:  giremi -f hg19.fa -l test.txt -o RNAE.lst test_dup.bam
```

The RNA editing sites are output into the list file "RNAE.lst".

3. Description of the GIREMI results

The output file of GIREMI includes a rich list of information about the SNVs. The columns are briefly explained as below:

(a) chr: Chromosome or scaffold identification.

(b) coordinate: Position of the SNVs in the chromosome or scaffold (1-based).

(c) strand: Strand information.

(d) ifSNP: 1, If the SNV is included in dbSNP; 0: otherwise.

(e) gene: Name of the gene harboring this SNV.

(f) reference_base: The nucleotide of this SNV in the reference chromosome (+ strand).

(g) upstream_1base: The upstream neighboring nucleotide of this SNV in the reference chromosome (+ strand).

(h) downstream_1base: The downstream neighboring nucleotide of this SNV in the reference chromosome (+ strand).

(i) major_base: The major nucleotide of the SNV in the RNA-seq data.

(j) major_count: Number of reads with the major nucleotide.

(k) tot_count: Total number of reads covering this SNV in the RNA-Seq data.

(l)   major_ratio: The ratio of major nucleotide (major_count/tot_count).

(m)   MI: The mutual information of this SNV if a value exists.

(n)   pvalue_mi: P-value from the MI test if applicable.

(o)   estimated_allelic_ratio: Estimated allelic ratio of the gene harboring this SNV.

(p)   ifNEG: 1: this SNV was a negative control in the training data.

(q)   RNAE_t: Type of RNA editing or RNA-DNA mismatches (A-to-G etc.).

(r)   A, C, G, T: Numbers of reads with specific nucleotides at this site.

(s)   ifRNAE: 1: the SNV is predicted as an RNA editing site based on MI analysis; 2: the SNV is predicted as an RNA editing site based on GLM 0: the SNV is not predicted as an RNA editing site.

4   Notes

1. GIREMI starts to predict the RNA-editing sites from a list of credible SNVs with known SNPs and the corresponding bam file. The users must do the alignment and call SNVs using the external tools. As we have discussed, GIREMI is sensitive to the errors from sequencing, PCR or other sources. So the stringent rules are required to remove these errors as much as possible. Previously, we used a "double filters" scheme to maximize mapping rate while maintaining high mapping accuracy [13]. This scheme, called "obviously best" filtering scheme now, has been adopted by RASER [21], an alignment software superbly efficient in unbiased mapping of the alternative alleles of SNPs and in identification of RNA editing sites. Other filters could also be further applied to remove potential artifacts resulted from sequencing or mapping bias.

2. GIREMI also accepts the bam file and SNVs list from other alignment and SNV calling tools. The user should make sure the bam file is the exact one from which the SNVs are called since some software tools may generate many intermediate bam files. GIREMI uses the pileup way to collect all kinds of information of each SNV same to samtools, so the variant frequency might be slightly different from that generated by GATK in some cases.

3. As introduced in Subheading 3, GIREMI firstly uses the distribution of MI of the known SNP pairs to judge whether a SNV with MI value is a RNA editing site. The user should only mark the high confidential SNPs, otherwise the error-marked SNPs

might shift the distribution to smaller value and increase the false positive. GIREMI prints the mean and variance of the MI distribution on the screen. In theory, the mean should be 0.69. However, because of the sequencing depth and reads length, we cannot build the ideal distribution all the time. So the mean value usually is around 0.6. If the mean of MI is smaller than 0.5, there may be too many sequencing errors or RNA editing sites incorrectly marked as known SNPs.

4. Our experimental results showed that the false discovery rate (FDR) of GIREMI was only 7.6% even if the 90% unknown SNVs were SNPs. So the users need not worry about the composition of the unknown SNVs. In addition, GIREMI is not sensitive to the single-end or pair-end reads. The low sequencing depth can decrease the total detectable SNVs, but does not affect the FDR of GIREMI.

5. All the SNVs are reported in the final result file, and only those with nonzero "ifRNAE" sites are predicted as RNA editing sites.

References

1. Keegan LP, Gallo A, O'Connell MA (2001) The many roles of an RNA editor. Nat Rev Genet 2:869–878

2. Wang Q, Miyakoda M, Yang W et al (2004) Stress-induced apoptosis associated with null mutation of ADAR1 RNA editing deaminase gene. J Biol Chem 279:4952–4961

3. Higuchi M, Maas S, Single FN et al (2000) Point mutation in an AMPA receptor gene rescues lethality in mice deficient in the RNA-editing enzyme ADAR2. Nature 406:78–81

4. Maas S, Kawahara Y, Tamburro KM, Nishikura K (2006) A-to-I RNA editing and human disease. RNA Biol 3:1–9

5. Miyamura Y, Suzuki T, Kono M, Inagaki K, Ito S, Suzuki N et al (2003) Mutations of the RNA-specific adenosine deaminase gene (DSRAD) are involved in dyschromatosis symmetrica hereditaria. Am J Hum Genet 73:693–699

6. Rice GI, Kasher PR, Forte GM, Mannion NM, Greenwood SM, Szynkiewicz M et al (2012) Mutations in ADAR1 cause Aicardi-Goutieres syndrome associated with a type I interferon signature. Nat Genet 44:1243–1248

7. Chen L (2013) Characterization and comparison of human nuclear and cytosolic editomes. Proc Natl Acad Sci U S A 110:E2741–E2747

8. Paz N, Levanon EY, Amariglio N, Heimberger AB, Ram Z, Constantini S et al (2007) Altered adenosine-to-inosine RNA editing in human cancer. Genome Res 17:1586–1595

9. Paz-Yaacov N, Bazak L, Buchumenski I, Porath HT, Danan-Gotthold M, Knisbacher BA et al (2015) Elevated RNA editing activity is a major contributor to transcriptomic diversity in tumors. Cell Rep 13:267–276

10. Han L, Diao L, Yu S, Xu X, Li J, Zhang R et al (2015) The genomic landscape and clinical relevance of A-to-I RNA editing in human cancers. Cancer Cell 28:515–528

11. Lee J-H, Ang JK, Xiao X (2013) Analysis and design of RNA sequencing experiments for identifying RNA editing and other single-nucleotide variants. RNA 19:725–732

12. Ramaswami G, Zhang R, Piskol R, Keegan LP, Deng P, O'Connell MA, Li JB (2013) Identifying RNA editing sites using RNA sequencing data alone. Nat Methods 10:128–132

13. Zhang Q, Xiao X (2015) Genome sequence-independent identification of RNA editing sites. Nat Methods 12:347–350

14. Langmead B, Trapnell C, Pop M, Salzberg SL (2009) Ultrafast and memory-efficient alignment of short DNA sequences to the human genome. Genome Biol 10:R25

15. Li H, Durbin R (2009) Fast and accurate short read alignment with Burrows-Wheeler Transform. Bioinformatics 25:1754–1760

16. Kent WJ (2002) BLAT--the BLAST-like alignment tool. Genome Res 12(4):656–664

17. McKenna A, Hanna M, Banks E, Sivachenko A, Cibulskis K, Kernytsky A, Garimella K, Altshuler D, Gabriel S, Daly M, DePristo MA (2010) The genome analysis toolkit: a MapReduce framework for analyzing next-generation DNA sequencing data. Genome Res 20:1297–1303

18. DePristo M, Banks E, Poplin R, Garimella K, Maguire J, Hartl C, Philippakis A, del Angel G, Rivas MA, Hanna M, McKenna A, Fennell T, Kernytsky A, Sivachenko A, Cibulskis K, Gabriel S, Altshuler D, Daly M (2011) A framework for variation discovery and genotyping using next-generation DNA sequencing data. Nat Genet 43:491–498

19. Van der Auwera GA, Carneiro M, Hartl C, Poplin R, del Angel G, Levy-Moonshine A, Jordan T, Shakir K, Roazen D, Thibault J, Banks E, Garimella K, Altshuler D, Gabriel S, DePristo M (2013) From FastQ data to high-confidence variant calls: the genome analysis toolkit best practices pipeline. Curr Protoc Bioinformatics 43:11.10.1–11.10.33

20. Li H (2011) A statistical framework for SNP calling, mutation discovery, association mapping and population genetical parameter estimation from sequencing data. Bioinformatics 27(21):2987–2993

21. Ahn J, Xiao X (2015) RASER: reads aligner for SNPs and editing sites of RNA. Bioinformatics 31(24):3906–3913

Chapter 8

Bioinformatic Analysis of MicroRNA Sequencing Data

Xiaonan Fu and Daoyuan Dong

Abstract

The vital role of microRNAs (miRNAs) involved in gene expression regulation has been confirmed in many biological processes. With the growing power and reducing cost of next-generation sequencing, more and more researchers turn to apply this high-throughput method to solve their biological problems. For miRNAs with known sequences, their expression profiles can be generated from the sequencing data. It also allows us to identify some novel miRNAs and explore the sequence variations under different conditions. Currently, there are a handful of tools available to analyze the miRNA sequencing data with separated or combined features, such as reads preprocessing, mapping and differential expression analysis. However, to our knowledge, a hands-on guideline for miRNA sequencing data analysis covering all steps is not available. Here we will utilize a set of published tools to perform the miRNA analysis with detailed explanation. Particularly, the miRNA target prediction and annotation may provide useful information for further experimental verification.

Key words MicroRNAs, miRNAs, Bioinformatic, R, mirPRo, Small RNA sequencing

1 Introduction

MicroRNAs (miRNAs) are small noncoding RNAs with size around 22 nt [1]. The biogenesis of miRNAs is mainly associated with two RNase III proteins—Drosha and Dicer [2]. Guided by mature miRNA, the Argonaute (Ago) protein forms a complex with miRNA to regulate the targeting gene expression [3]. With these features, miRNA libraries are generally prepared from total RNAs by size selection or associated protein immunoprecipitation (IP) such as Ago-IP. Commercialized kits designed for small RNA libraries generated in different scenarios are available to adapt to various platforms [4]. To produce a reliable dataset, the experimental strategy should be carefully chosen since bias could be introduced in multiple steps during library construction such as adapter ligation [5]. The high quality profile of miRNAs is a good start of the project.

Typically, the bioinformatic analysis of miRNA sequencing data consists of five parts: (1) Data preprocessing, including reads

Yejun Wang and Ming-an Sun (eds.), *Transcriptome Data Analysis: Methods and Protocols*, Methods in Molecular Biology, vol. 1751, https://doi.org/10.1007/978-1-4939-7710-9_8, © Springer Science+Business Media, LLC 2018

quality filtering and 3′-adapter trimming; (2) Reads mapping and annotation; (3) Sequence feature analysis, including novel miRNA prediction and the analysis of sequence variation of mature miRNAs isoforms; (4) Differential expression analysis, regarding both known and novel miRNAs; (5) Functional analysis, based on miRNA target prediction. Currently, there are a number of tools providing one or more modules for analyzing the miRNA sequencing data. Hereinbefore, several tools have been developed integrating multiple programs into a single pipeline such as mirTools [6, 7], mirPRo [8], CAP-miRSeq [9], miARma-Seq [10], and Chimira [11]. Except for the web-based Chimira, the others are stand-alone tool suites, which can be downloaded, and run locally. Here, we have chosen mirPRo combining with fastx toolkit, flexbar [12], TargetScan [13, 14], and miRBase [15–18] to describe their use in miRNA sequencing analysis. Particularly, the selection of mirPRo is because it incorporates almost all the modules for analyzing miRNA sequencing data. In addition, the integrated tools in mirPRo, including mirDeep [19] and RNAfold [20], have been widely used in many miRNAs studies. In this protocol, we will use the sample dataset from a MCF7 cell line study to demonstrate the bioinformatic analysis of miRNA sequencing data [21].

2   Materials

1. Hardware: Linux or Mac OS system is required to install the software. Computer requirement depends on the size of the dataset. Generally, a regular PC is enough for the analysis. For this tutorial, the analysis was run on a 64-bit computer with 32 GB of RAM and 16 CPUs installed with Linux system Ubuntu 15.10.

2. All the commands in this protocol have been tested in the Linux system. If rerun the same analysis, make sure that all the required files are in the working directory. Commands executed under the Linux terminal are prefixed with a "$" character. Commands executed in the R console are prefixed with a ">" character. All the outputs are prefixed with a "##" character.

3. miRNA sequencing datasets (accession GSE47602 at Gene Expression Omnibus of NCBI): Datasets downloaded from NCBI Gene Expression Omnibus (https://www.ncbi.nlm.nih.gov/geo/) with accession GSE47602 were downloaded for demonstration. To download the dataset, go to the website and search by the accession number (Con1: SRR873382; Con2: SRR873383; Exp1: SRR873384; Exp2: SRR873385). Alternatively, open the terminal and download through the wget command (e.g., wget ftp://ftp-trace.ncbi.nlm.nih.gov/sra/sra-instant/reads/ByExp/sra/SRX/SRX290/SRX290631/

SRR873382/SRR873382.sra). The datasets should be down-loaded one by one and then renamed for each experiment.

4. Database files: Several reference and annotation files (known miRNA sequence, GTF file for gene annotation, genome sequence) are required in this protocol. The sequence files (mature.fa.gz, hairpin.fa.gz) for known miRNAs can be downloaded from the miRBase ftp site (ftp://mirbase.org/pub/mirbase/CURRENT/). The reference genome and gene annotation files (Homo_sapiens.GRCh38.dna.primary_assembly.fa.gz, Homo_sapiens.GRCh38.81.gtf.gz) can be downloaded from the Ensembl database (ftp://ftp.ensembl.org/pub/release-81/fasta/homo_sapiens/, ftp://ftp.ensembl.org/pub/release-81/gtf/homo_sapiens/).

5. Software installation: The software used in this protocol can be downloaded from their websites as below:

sra-toolkits (https://github.com/ncbi/sra-tools); fastx_toolkit (http://hannonlab.cshl.edu/fastx_toolkit); Flexbar (https://github.com/seqan/flexbar); RNAfold (http://www.tbi.univie.ac.at/RNA); randfold (http://bioinformatics.psb.ugent.be/supplementary_data/erbon/nov2003/); Novoalign (http://www.novocraft.com/support/download/); HTSeq (http://www-huber.embl.de/users/anders/HTSeq/); mirPRo (https://sourceforge.net/p/mirpro); rstudio (https://www.rstudio.com/products/rstudio/download/). Download the tools from the corresponding website to your software directory. All the tools provide installation guide. Once finishing setting up, you should run the command (export PATH=$PATH:your-directory/your-tools/) in order to access the tools directly from the terminal.

6. Install the R package for the later analysis.
Open the Rstudio and run the following scripts to install the required packages.

```
>source("https://bioconductor.org/biocLite.R")
>biocLite("DESeq2")
>install.packages("pheatmap")
```

3 Methods

3.1 Environment Setup

1. Open the terminal and create a working directory.

```
$mkdir working-directory
```

2. Move the sequencing files and database files into the working directory and check their status

```
$ls
##SRR873382.sra
##SRR873383.sra
##SRR873384.sra
##SRR873385.sra
##mature.fa.gz
##hairpin.fa.gz
##Homo_sapiens.GRCh38.dna.primary_assembly.fa.gz
##Homo_sapiens.GRCh38.81.gtf.gz
```

3. Convert the .sra files into .fastq files and decompress the .gz files.

```
$fastq-dump *.sra
$gunzip *.gz
```

4. Rename the fastq files.

```
$mv SRR873382.fastq Con1.fastq
$mv SRR873383.fastq Con2.fastq
$mv SRR873384.fastq Exp1.fastq
$mv SRR873385.fastq Exp2.fastq
```

3.2 Preprocessing

A fastq sequencing files should consist of four lines per read. The first line starts with "@" followed by the sequence identifier. The second line is the raw sequence letters, with undetermined nucleotide appearing as "N." The third line has "+" as the first character optionally had the same header information as the first line. The fourth line is the base quality value for the raw sequence. The raw sequence files need to be preprocessed to filter out the reads of bad quality. As for miRNA sequencing data, the 3′-adapter trimming has to be performed due to the short length of miRNAs.

1. Remove the reads of bad quality using *fastq_quality_filter* from fastx-toolkit. Option "q" is the minimum quality score to keep. Option "p" is minimum percent of bases for each read with sequencing score higher than "q."

```
$fastq_quality_filter -q 20 -p 95 -i Con1.fastq -o Con1_qf.
fastq
$fastq_quality_filter -q 20 -p 95 -i Con2.fastq -o Con2_qf.
fastq
$fastq_quality_filter -q 20 -p 95 -i Exp1.fastq -o Exp1_qf.
fastq
$fastq_quality_filter -q 20 -p 95 -i Exp2.fastq -o Exp2_qf.
fastq
```

2. Trim the 3′-adapter with *flexbar*. Set the minimum overlap between read sequence and adapter sequence as 4 nt with option "ao." Only keep the reads with no less than 16 nt with option "m." The number of threads used for parallel computation was enabled with option "n."

```
$flexbar -t Con1_trimed -r Con1_qf.fastq -as ATCTCG-
TATGCCGTCTTCTGCTT -ao 4 -m 16 -n 6
$flexbar -t Con2_trimed -r Con2_qf.fastq -as ATCTCG-
TATGCCGTCTTCTGCTT -ao 4 -m 16 -n 6
$flexbar -t Exp1_trimed -r Exp1_qf.fastq -as ATCTCG-
TATGCCGTCTTCTGCTT -ao 4 -m 16 -n 6
$flexbar -t Exp2_trimed -r Exp2_qf.fastq -as ATCTCG-
TATGCCGTCTTCTGCTT -ao 4 -m 16 -n 6
```

3. Get the length distribution of total reads to have an overview of the datasets.

```
$cat Con1_trimed.fastq | awk '{if(NR%4==2) print length
($1)}' | sort -n | uniq -c >Con1_readLength.txt
$cat Con2_trimed.fastq | awk '{if(NR%4==2) print length
($1)}' | sort -n | uniq -c >Con2_readLength.txt
$cat Exp1_trimed.fastq | awk '{if(NR%4==2) print length
($1)}' | sort -n | uniq -c >Exp1_readLength.txt
$cat Exp2_trimed.fastq | awk '{if(NR%4==2) print length
($1)}' | sort -n | uniq -c >Exp2_readLength.txt
```

4. Open the Rstudio. The R command should be run in the left panel (Fig. 1a). The figures will be produced in the right panel (Fig. 1b).

5. Setup the working directory and load the data from step 3. Using the *head()* function to check the loaded datasets, there are two columns for each dataset: the first column is frequency and the second column is read length.

```
>setwd("~/your-working-directory")
>Con1_lengthDis = read.table("Con1_readLength.txt")
>Con2_lengthDis = read.table("Con2_readLength.txt")
>Exp1_lengthDis = read.table("Exp1_readLength.txt")
>Exp2_lengthDis = read.table("Exp2_readLength.txt")
>head(Con1_lengthDis)## V1 V2
##1 232515 16
##2 325012 17
##3 308513 18
##4 294719 19
##5 485567 20
##6 1803169 21
```

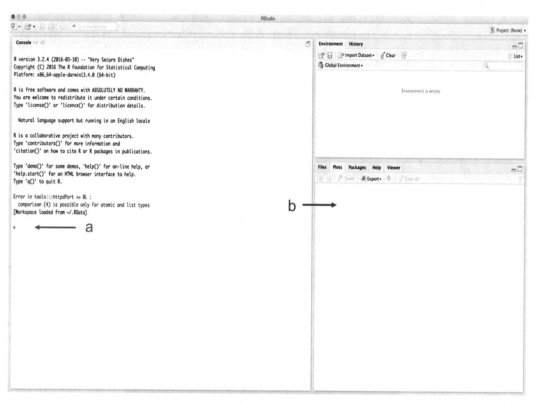

Fig. 1 The Rstudio interface. Rstudio is an R language IDE for statistical analysis and graphics

6. Produce the figures of reads length distribution. The read length might vary in different datasets. We choose to focus on 16–30 nt which corresponds to row 1–15 of the dataset. Control group (Fig. 2a) and experimental group (Fig. 2b) were plotted separately with different color schemes. The most abundant peak is 23 nt for both groups. Similar distribution was observed between the two groups with most reads ranged from 21 to 24 nt. These patterns suggest the enriched miRNAs from sequencing data.

```
>ConColor = c("gray20","gray70")
>ExpColor = c("pink","red")
>barplot(rbind(Con1_lengthDis[1:15,1],Con2_lengthDis
[1:15,1])/1000000,names.arg = 16:30,beside = T,col=ConCo-
lor,ylab="Total read counts (M)",xlab="Adapter trimed reads
length",main = "Length Distribution")
>legend("topleft",c("Con1","Con2"),bty="n",fill = ConCo-
lor)
>barplot(rbind(Exp1_lengthDis[1:15,1],Exp2_lengthDis
[1:15,1])/1000000,names.arg = 16:30, beside= T,col=ExpCo-
lor,ylab="Total read counts(M)",xlab="Adapter trimed reads
```

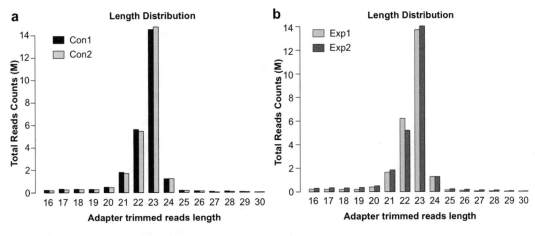

Fig. 2 The length distribution of total sequenced reads. The length of clean raw reads for control group (**a**) and experimental group (**b**) is plotted against their frequency

```
length",main = "Length Distribution")
>legend("topleft",c("Exp1","Exp2"),bty="n",fill  =  ExpCo-
lor)
```

3.3 mirPRo Pipeline

The mirPRo stand-alone pipeline is capable of genome mapping, known miRNAs annotation, novel miRNAs identification, and arm switching detection. These results can be produced from one command line.

1. Create the genome index file using *novoindex* from preinstalled novoalign.

```
$novoindex hg38.idx Homo_sapiens.GRCh38.dna.primary_assem-
bly.fa
##novoindex (3.7) - Universal k-mer index constructor.
##(C) 2008 - 2011 NovoCraft Technologies SdnBhd
##novoindex hg39.idx Homo_sapiens.GRCh38.dna.primary_assem-
bly.fa
##Creating 24 indexing threads.
##Building with 14-mer and step of 2 bp.
```

2. Run the pipeline using preprocessed data. The options for quality filtering and adapter trimming is disabled by "-a 0" and "-q 0" since the input is clean reads. The option "-s hsa" is specified for human species. If the dataset is from other species, the three-letter code of the corresponding species can be obtained from miRBase. The human GTF file is provided to annotate other RNA classes. Novel miRNA identification is enabled with "--novel 1". The option "-other" is set as "mmu" for identification of conserved seed between different species (human and mouse

in this case). The pipeline is run in parallel model with "-t 4". It takes about two hours for the sample data.

```
$mirpro -i Con1_trimed.fastq -i Con2_trimed.fastq -i Ex-
p1_trimed.fastq -i Exp2_trimed.fastq -m mature.fa -p hair-
pin.fa -d ./miRNA -s hsa -a 0 -q 0 -t 4 --gtf Homo_sapiens.
GRCh38.81.gtf --novel 1 --other mmu -g Homo_sapiens.GRCh38.
dna.primary_assembly.fa --index hg38.idx
#start:
#checking prerequisite programs ...
#checking parameters ...
#processing known mature miRNA and precursor miRNA data...
```

3. Interpret the output of mirPRo. The clean reads are first mapped to miRNAs. The detailed mapping information is stored under /miRNA/result/sample/*_mature_miRNA_mapping.csv. The structure of this file is organized in multiple sequence alignment format (Fig. 3). The remaining sequencing reads are then mapped to the genome. The mapping results are outputted as /miRNA/run/sample/*_vs_genome_t_60_count.sam. The final results for the whole analysis can be found in the directory of /miRNA/result/. The count number of known and novel miRNAs is in the file "result_mature.csv" and "result_novel_-mature.csv". Other processed files are also included. The file

```
hsa-mir-188 ← a  NA    NA b → ugcucccucucucacaucccuugcaugguggagggugagcuuucugaaaaccccucccacaugcaggguuugcaggauggcgagcc
hsa-miR-188-5p   NA    NA     ..............caucccuugcaugguggaggg ← c...................................................
hsa-miR-188-3p   NA  e NA     .....................................................cucccacaugcaggguuugca............
80731-2 ← d      2 ← 0/0/0/0  ..............caucccuugcaugguggaUGGA..................................................
13941-16         16   0/0/0/0  ..............caucccuugcauggugga......................................................
84525-2          2    0/0/0/0  ..............caucccuugcaugguggagA....................................................
131742-1         1    0/0/0/0  ..............caucccuugcaugguggagAU...................................................
501746-1         1    1/0/0/0  ..............caucccuugcCugguggag.....................................................
150746-1         1    1/0/0/0  ..............caucccuugcaugAuggag.....................................................
5675-55          55   0/0/0/0  ..............caucccuugcaugguggag.....................................................
588928-1         1    1/0/0/0  ..............caucccuugcauAguggaggA...................................................
508402-1         1    0/0/0/0  ..............caucccuugcaugguggaggGUAGU...............................................
392533-1         1    0/0/0/0  ..............caucccuugcaugguggaggAA..................................................
28918-6          6    1/0/0/0  ..............caucccuugcCugguggagg....................................................
255993-1         1    0/0/0/0  ..............caucccuugcaugguggaggAUU.................................................
244654-1         1    1/0/0/0  ..............caucccuugcaugguAgagg....................................................
63352-3          3    0/0/0/0  ..............caucccuugcaugguggaggA...................................................
1408-395         395  0/0/0/0  ..............caucccuugcaugguggagg....................................................
212388-1         1    0/0/0/0  ..............caucccuugcaugguggagggUUG................................................
5562-57          57   0/0/0/0  ..............caucccuugcaugguggaggg...................................................
51343-3          3    0/0/0/0  ..............caucccuugcaugguggagggA..................................................
193040-1         1    0/0/0/0  ..............caucccuugcaugguggagggAAU................................................
110320-2         2    0/0/0/0  ..............caucccuugcaugguggaggguAG................................................
458046-1         1    0/0/0/0  ..............caucccuugcaugguggaggguUAGA..............................................
44544-4          4    0/0/0/0  ..............caucccuugcaugguggaggguA.................................................
220989-1         1    0/0/0/0  ..............caucccuugcaugguggaggguAGG...............................................
21916-9          9    0/0/0/0  ..............caucccuugcaugguggaggguU.................................................
13555-17         17   0/0/0/0  ..............caucccuugcaugguggagggu..................................................
124780-2         2    0/0/0/0  ..............caucccuugcaugguggagggug.................................................
290364-1         1    0/0/0/0  .....................................................cucccacaugcaggguuugc.............
423386-1         1    0/0/0/0  .....................................................cucccacaugcaggguuugca............
```

Fig. 3 Mapping of sequencing reads back to miRNA precursor for mir-188. (**a**) Name of miRNA precursor. (**b**) Hairpin sequence of miRNA precursor. (**c**) Mature miRNA sequence. (**d**) ID of collapsed sequencing reads. (**e**) Count number of the sequencing read

"3_other_form.csv" consists of statistics for the mature miRNA 3'-end variation. The mapping statistics and RNA catalog information are contained in "read_cataloging.csv". The predicted novel miRNA sequences are stored in "novel_mature.fa" and "novel_precursor.fa".

4. Summarize the read mapping information. This result will be loaded into R for exploration.

   (a) Load the file into Rstudio. Exclude the first two empty lines by 'skip =2'.

   ```
   >annotation = as.matrix(read.csv("final/result/read_-
   cataloging.csv",header=T,row.names = 1,skip=2))
   ```

   (b) Change the name of columns to the sample names and remove the lines start with "__". These four lines are overall mapping summary, which do not belong to any RNA category.

   ```
   >colnames(annotation) = c("Con1","Con2","Exp1","Exp2")
   >remove = c("__alignment_not_unique", "__ambi-
   guous","__no_feature","__not_aligned")
   >annotation = annotation[!(rownames(annotation) %in%
   remove),]
   ```

   (c) Remove the lines with empty read mapping, and check the final results of read mapping.

   ```
   >annotation = annotation[rowMax(annotation)>0,]
   >annotation
   #  Con1 Con2 Exp1 Exp2
   #Mt_rRNA  3140 2772 3252 3016
   #Mt_tRNA  7719 5997 9223 8665
   #antisense  2232 1765 876 1419
   #lincRNA  1155 1231 954 1126
   #miRNA 4077316 3834806 3445130 3783094
   #misc_RNA 1203 1423 452 516
   #processed_pseudogene 420 336 371 399
   #processed_transcript 34342 26672 11114 43866
   #protein_coding  58624 50793 37678 48743
   #sense_intronic 262 388 122 146
   #snRNA  984 981 407 659
   #snoRNA  20812 1 5821 9162 27440
   ```

3.4 Novel miRNA Prediction

The novel miRNA prediction is performed by mirDeep2. This tool is integrated into the mirPRo pipeline. For the sample dataset, there are 509 novel miRNAs. The miRNA hairpin structure can be checked with *RNAfold* as follows.

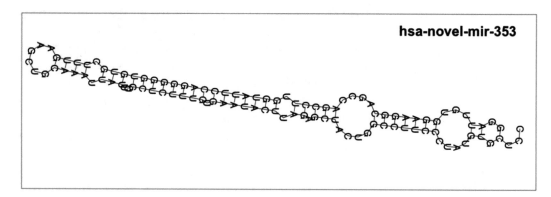

Fig. 4 RNA secondary structure of novel-mir-353 from RNAfold

1. Extract the novel miRNA precursor sequences from the file "novel_precursor.fa". For example, hsa-novel-mir-353:

```
$cat novel_precursor.fa | awk '$1==">hsa-mir-353"{print;
getline;print}' >novelmir353.fa
```

2. Run RNAfold with the novel-mir-353 precursor sequence. The output in the terminal is a RNA secondary structure of minimum free energy in dot-bracket interaction pattern. The dot represents unpaired nucleotide whereas the parentheses are paired positions. There is also a figure of secondary structure generated under the working directory (Fig. 4).

```
$RNAfold <novelmir353.fa
##>hsa-novel-mir-353 3:-:33925657:33925764
##GGAUUGUGGAAGGCAGCCAGCCUUGGUAUUCCAGGGGGUGUGCUUUGAAGCUG-
CAAAUUAUUUGCUCUUUGUGAAUACUUAGAGCUACUGGCCUUCCCUAUGUGCUCC
##(.((...((((((((....(((((.((((((((((((((((((((.
(((((......)))).)))...)))))))))).)))))))).)).))).....)))))))...-
.)).)... (-37.00)
```

3.5 Differentially Expressed miRNAs

The identification of differentially expressed miRNAs is performed by R package DESeq2 [22]. The raw read count number of known and novel miRNAs will be combined as a single input for DESeq2. With the default setting, normalized read counts will be used for comparison. The adjusted p-value < 0.1 based on negative binomial distribution is considered statistically significant.

1. Open the Rstudio and install the Bioconductor package DESeq2 and its dependences by running the following scripts. Install the R package pheatmap for the later analysis.

```
>source("https://bioconductor.org/biocLite.R")
>biocLite("DESeq2")
>install.packages("pheatmap")
>library("DESeq2")
>library("pheatmap")
```

2. Load the miRNA quantification file into Rstudio. Exclude the first two empty lines by 'skip =2'.

```
>known=as.matrix(read.csv("final/result/result_mature.
csv",row.names="id",skip=2))
>novel=as.matrix(read.csv("final/result/result_novel_ma-
ture.csv",row.names="id",skip=2))
```

3. Organize the count matrix. The known and novel miRNAs are combined into one matrix.

```
>miRNA = rbind(known,novel) #combine the known and novel
miRNAs
>colnames(miRNA) = c("Con1","Con2","Exp1","Exp2")
```

4. Create the experimental setting table. The samples "Con1" and "Con2" are in the group of "Con" and the samples "Exp1" and "Exp2" are in the group of "Exp".

```
>expsetting<- data.frame(condition=factor(rep(c("Con","-
Exp"),each=2)))
>rownames(expsetting) <- colnames(miRNA)
>expsetting
## condition
##Con1 Con
##Con2 Con
##Exp1 Exp
##Exp2 Exp
```

5. Load the data into DESeq2. Prefilter the data to remove miR-NAs that have only 0 or 1 read. Run the differential expression analysis with default setting.

```
>mirnaDeseq=DESeqDataSetFromMatrix(countData = miRNA,col-
Data = expsetting,design = ~ condition)
>mirnaDeseq =mirnaDeseq [rowSums(counts(mirnaDeseq)) > 1,]
>mirnaDeseq = DESeq(mirnaDeseq)
```

6. Check the results from DESeq2 and the explanations for six columns are as follows.

```
>result<- results(mirnaDeseq)
>result
##log2 fold change (MAP): condition Expvs Con
##Wald test p-value: condition Expvs Con
##DataFrame with 1865 rows and 6 columns
##baseMean log2FoldChange lfcSE stat pvaluepadj
##<numeric><numeric><numeric><numeric><numeric><numeri-
c>
##hsa-let-7a-3p  6.569788e+02  -0.4453378  0.3430238
-1.2982708 0.1941943 0.999521
##hsa-let-7a-5p 1.517097e+06 0.3565467 0.3549906 1.0043834
0.3151938 0.999521
##hsa-let-7b-3p  8.425011e+01  -0.6053872  0.4041295
-1.4980029 0.1341325 0.999521
##hsa-let-7b-5p  4.699590e+05  -0.2545546  0.3644794
-0.6984058 0.4849234 0.999521
##hsa-let-7c-3p  2.442498e+01  -0.3501618  0.4584878
-0.7637320 0.4450269 0.999521
>mcols(result)$description
##[1] "mean of normalized counts for all samples"
##[2] "log2 fold change (MAP): condition Exp vs Con"
##[3] "standard error: condition Exp vs Con"
##[4] "Wald statistic: condition Exp vs Con"
##[5] "Wald test p-value: condition Exp vs Con"
##[6] "BH adjusted p-values"
```

7. Explore the differentially expressed miRNAs in the result. Through the "summary" function, we know there are 1865 miRNAs with nonzero total count. Four upregulated miRNAs and five downregulated miRNAs are identified.

```
>summary(result)
##out of 1865 with nonzero total read count
##adjusted p-value < 0.1
##LFC > 0 (up) : 4, 0.21%
##LFC < 0 (down) : 5, 0.27%
##outliers [1] : 0, 0%
##low counts [2] : 0, 0%
##(mean count < 0)
```

8. Present the result of differentially expressed (DE) miRNAs by MA plot (Fig. 5a) and heatmap (Fig. 5b). Output the DE miRNAs list into a file using "write.table" (*see* **Note 1**).

```
>plotMA(result, main="Differentially Expression miRNAs",
ylim=c(-2,2))
>mirnaresult = as.data.frame(result)
>diff = mirnaresult[mirnaresult$padj<0.1,]
```

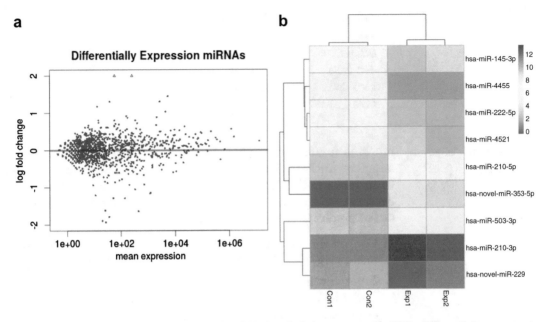

Fig. 5 Differentially expressed miRNAs. (**a**) The MA plot of all the expressed miRNAs. Differentially expressed (DE) miRNAs are in red. (**b**) The heatmap of DE miRNAs. Normalized counts were log2(count+1) transformed

```
>pheatmap(log2(miRNA_normalization[rownames(diff),]+1),
clustering_method = "single")
>write.table(diff,"DE_miRNA.txt")
```

3.6 miRNA 3′-End Variation

The strong homogeneity of miRNAs 5′end resulting from highly accurate cleavage by Drosha/Dicer has been confirmed in many species [23]. In this analysis, we will only focus on 3′-end nontemplate variation. This result is stored in the file "3_other_form.csv".

1. Load 3′-end nontemplate variation data into Rstudio. Exclude the first two empty lines by 'skip =2'.

```
>variation3 = as.matrix(read.csv("final/result/3_other_-
form.csv",header=T,row.names = 1,skip=2))
```

2. Show the top ten 3′-end nontemplate variations. The most frequent 3′-end variation is "A" addition.

```
>select = order(rowMeans(variation3),decreasing=TRUE)
[1:10]
>variation3[select,]
## Con1_trimed Con2_trimed Exp1_trimed Exp2_trimed
##A 211169 241810 256976 143374
##U 152834 173216 209556 139348
##AA 11536 16673 12818 7195
##G 11373 11076 8140 11198
```

```
##UU  6466    6975 7715 5412
##AU  6163    8783 5271 5526
##AG  4284    4434 2635 4491
##C   3191    3637 2919 2849
##UA  2718    3012 3388 2081
##AAA 2045    2569 1375 1006
```

3.7 miRNAs Target Prediction

miRNAs regulate the gene expression through interacting with targeting mRNAs. Defining the targets of miRNAs is a key step to understand the functional role of miRNAs. Nine miRNAs are detected abnormally expressed in this analysis. We will use TargetScan to predict their targets (*see* **Note 2**).

1. Choose the species of the sample origin from the drop-down menu (Fig. 6a). "human" is chosen in this analysis.

2. Input the name of the miRNA of your interest and submit. Hsa-miR-210-3p is upregulated, thus was shown here as an example in Table 1.

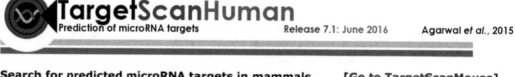

TargetScanHuman
Prediction of microRNA targets   Release 7.1: June 2016   *Agarwal et al., 2015*

Search for predicted microRNA targets in mammals   [Go to TargetScanMouse]
[Go to TargetScanWorm]
[Go to TargetScanFly]
[Go to TargetScanFish]

1. Select a species   Human   ◧ ⟵ a

AND

2. Enter a human gene symbol (e.g. "Hmga2")
   or an Ensembl gene (ENSG00000149948) or transcript (ENST00000403681) ID

AND/OR

3. Do one of the following:

• Select a broadly conserved* microRNA family Broadly conserved microRNA families ◧

• Select a conserved* microRNA family Conserved microRNA families ◧

• Select a poorly conserved but confidently annotated microRNA family Poorly conserved microRNA families ◧

• Select another miRBase annotation Other miRBase annotations
Note that most of these families are star miRNAs or RNA fragments misannotated as miRNAs.

• Enter a microRNA name (e.g. "miR-9-5p") hsa-mir-210-3p ⟵ b

Submit   Reset

* broadly conserved = conserved across most vertebrates, usually to zebrafish
conserved = conserved across most mammals, but usually not beyond placental mammals

Fig. 6 TargetScan for miRNAs target prediction (http:/www.targetscan.org/vert_71/)

Table 1
List of predicted targets for hsa-miR-210-3p

Target gene	Representative transcript	Conserved sites
FGFRL1	ENST00000264748.6	7
ISCU	ENST00000338291.4	1
SCARA3	ENST00000301904.3	2
DIMT1	ENST00000199320.4	1
ST3GAL3	ENST00000372377.4	1
FAM89B	ENST00000449319.2	1
ELFN2	ENST00000402918.2	1
B4GALT5	ENST00000371711.4	1
DENND6A	ENST00000311128.5	1
FAM73B	ENST00000358369.4	1
AC137932.1	ENST00000602042.1	1
MEX3B	ENST00000558133.1	1
NDUFA4	ENST00000339600.5	1
EFNA3	ENST00000368408.3	1
SYNGAP1	ENST00000418600.2	1
CYGB	ENST00000293230.5	1
KMT2D	ENST00000301067.7	1
USP6NL	ENST00000609104.1	1
BDNF	ENST00000439476.2	1
E2F3	ENST00000346618.3	1
GPD1L	ENST00000282541.5	1
ZNF462	ENST00000277225.5	1
PPTC7	ENST00000354300.3	1
MID1IP1	ENST00000336949.6	1
BAZ2B	ENST00000392782.1	1
SEPT8	ENST00000378706.1	1
RAP2B	ENST00000323534.2	1
CDIP1	ENST00000564828.1	1
AC010327.2	ENST00000598855.1	1
DTX1	ENST00000257600.3	1
CPEB2	ENST00000538197.1	1

(continued)

Table 1
(continued)

Target gene	Representative transcript	Conserved sites
MEF2A	ENST00000354410.5	1
TET2	ENST00000545826.1	1
KLF7	ENST00000309446.6	1
CLUH	ENST00000570628.2	1
HIF3A	ENST00000377670.4	1
EFNA3	ENST00000505139.1	1
CELF2	ENST00000315874.4	1
ZNF74	ENST00000357502.5	1
KCMF1	ENST00000409785.4	1
NFIX	ENST00000360105.4	1
PCYT2	ENST00000538936.2	1
ATG7	ENST00000354449.3	1

3. A list of genes is output as potential targets of selected miRNA. Further experimental and functional studies are expected to validate the interaction of the miRNA–mRNA pair.

4 Notes

1. The normalized reads are log-transformed to generate the heatmap. To avoid zero logarithms, a pseudo value of 1 will be added before the calculation.

2. TargetScan includes miRNAs targets prediction from a lot of model animals. If you can not find your interesting species, you may find them in the miRanda [24] (http://www.microrna.org/microrna/home.do). Or you can run the miRNA target prediction following the guide of RNAhybrid [25] (https://bibiserv2.cebitec.uni-bielefeld.de/rnahybrid).

References

1. He L, Hannon GJ (2004) MicroRNAs: small RNAs with a big role in gene regulation. Nat Rev Genet 5(7):522–531

2. Kim VN, Han J, Siomi MC (2009) Biogenesis of small RNAs in animals. Nat Rev Mol Cell Biol 10(2):126–139

3. Siomi H, Siomi MC (2010) Posttranscriptional regulation of microRNA biogenesis in animals. Mol Cell 38(3):323–332

4. Baran-Gale J et al (2015) Addressing bias in small RNA library preparation for sequencing: a new protocol recovers MicroRNAs that evade capture by current methods. Front Genet 6:352

5. Fuchs RT et al (2015) Bias in ligation-based small RNA sequencing library construction is determined by adaptor and RNA structure. PLoS One 10(5):e0126049

6. Wu J et al (2013) mirTools 2.0 for non-coding RNA discovery, profiling, and functional annotation based on high-throughput sequencing. RNA Biol 10(7):1087–1092

7. Zhu E et al (2010) mirTools: microRNA profiling and discovery based on high-throughput sequencing. Nucleic Acids Res 38 (Web Server issue):W392–W397

8. Shi J et al (2015) mirPRo-a novel standalone program for differential expression and variation analysis of miRNAs. Sci Rep 5:14617

9. Sun Z et al (2014) CAP-miRSeq: a comprehensive analysis pipeline for microRNA sequencing data. BMC Genomics 15:423

10. Andres-Leon E, Nunez-Torres R, Rojas AM (2016) miARma-Seq: a comprehensive tool for miRNA, mRNA and circRNA analysis. Sci Rep 6:25749

11. Vitsios DM, Enright AJ (2015) Chimira: analysis of small RNA sequencing data and microRNA modifications. Bioinformatics 31 (20):3365–3367

12. Dodt M et al (2012) FLEXBAR-flexible barcode and adapter processing for next-generation sequencing platforms. Biology (Basel) 1(3):895–905

13. Agarwal V et al (2015) Predicting effective microRNA target sites in mammalian mRNAs. Elife 4:e05005

14. Lewis BP, Burge CB, Bartel DP (2005) Conserved seed pairing, often flanked by adenosines, indicates that thousands of human genes are microRNA targets. Cell 120 (1):15–20

15. Griffiths-Jones S (2006) miRBase: the microRNA sequence database. Methods Mol Biol 342:129–138

16. Griffiths-Jones S (2010) miRBase: microRNA sequences and annotation. Curr Protoc Bioinformatics Chapter 12:Unit 12 9 1–Unit 12 9 10

17. Kozomara A, Griffiths-Jones S (2011) miRBase: integrating microRNA annotation and deep-sequencing data. Nucleic Acids Res 39 (Database issue):152–157

18. Kozomara A, Griffiths-Jones S (2014) miRBase: annotating high confidence microRNAs using deep sequencing data. Nucleic Acids Res 42(Database issue):D68–D73

19. An J et al (2013) miRDeep*: an integrated application tool for miRNA identification from RNA sequencing data. Nucleic Acids Res 41(2):727–737

20. Lorenz R et al (2011) ViennaRNA package 2.0. Algorithms Mol Biol 6:26

21. Camps C et al (2014) Integrated analysis of microRNA and mRNA expression and association with HIF binding reveals the complexity of microRNA expression regulation under hypoxia. Mol Cancer 13:28

22. Love MI, Huber W, Anders S (2014) Moderated estimation of fold change and dispersion for RNA-seq data with DESeq2. Genome Biol 15(12):550

23. Shukla GC, Singh J, Barik S (2011) MicroRNAs: processing, maturation, target recognition and regulatory functions. Mol Cell Pharmacol 3(3):83–92

24. Enright AJ et al (2003) MicroRNA targets in Drosophila. Genome Biol 5(1):R1

25. Rehmsmeier M et al (2004) Fast and effective prediction of microRNA/target duplexes. RNA 10(10):1507–1517

Chapter 9

Microarray-Based MicroRNA Expression Data Analysis with Bioconductor

Emilio Mastriani, Rihong Zhai, and Songling Zhu

Abstract

MicroRNAs (miRNAs) are small, noncoding RNAs that are able to regulate the expression of targeted mRNAs. Thousands of miRNAs have been identified; however, only a few of them have been functionally annotated. Microarray-based expression analysis represents a cost-effective way to identify candidate miRNAs that correlate with specific biological pathways, and to detect disease-associated molecular signatures. Generally, microarray-based miRNA data analysis contains four major steps: (1) quality control and normalization, (2) differential expression analysis, (3) target gene prediction, and (4) functional annotation. For each step, a large couple of software tools or packages have been developed. In this chapter, we present a standard analysis pipeline for miRNA microarray data, assembled by packages mainly developed with *R* and hosted in Bioconductor project.

Key words MicroRNA (miRNA), Bioconcductor, R Package, Gene expression analysis, Microarray data analysis

1 Introduction

MicroRNAs (miRNAs) are small, noncoding and conserved RNA molecules that can inhibit protein expression by post-transcriptional regulation or translational repression. More than 20,000 different miRNAs have been disclosed among hundreds of species [1]. Although miRNAs play important roles in various biological processes, the function has only been well clarified for a small subset.

The expression profile of miRNAs often shows developmental stage or tissue specific patterns, suggesting that they may participate in the specific regulatory processes [2, 3]. Microarray is attractive to profile the miRNA expression under different conditions because it can detect thousands of miRNAs simultaneously [4]. Compared with other high-throughput technique, such as RNA-Seq, the cost of microarray-based studies appears much

Yejun Wang and Ming-an Sun (eds.), *Transcriptome Data Analysis: Methods and Protocols*, Methods in Molecular Biology, vol. 1751, https://doi.org/10.1007/978-1-4939-7710-9_9, © Springer Science+Business Media, LLC 2018

lower and hundreds or thousands of biological samples can be studied in one experiment with a cost-effective way.

There is some difference between the analytic pipelines of miRNA and other microarray-based expression data. Besides the routine preprocessing, expression comparison and functional annotation, miRNA data also involve additional target prediction and target gene annotation steps. For each step, a large number of bioinformatic tools have been developed. Experimental researchers will struggle to find, assemble and test the tools for the task of each step. In this chapter, we are going to present a pipeline specific for microarray-based miRNA expression data analysis. The pipeline is assembled by packages mostly hosted in Bioconductor project, and therefore all the analysis can be completed in *R* environment conveniently (R: http://www.r-project.org; Bioconductor: http://www.bioconductor.org).

2   Materials

2.1   Software Tools

2.1.1   R/Bioconductor

The most recent version of R was downloaded and installed. For this chapter, Linux platform is used. For R installation and administration, the FAQs and documents can be referred: https://www.r-project.org/. Bioconductor can be installed by entering the following commands after starting R:

```
> source("https://bioconductor.org/biocLite.R")
> biocLite()
```

2.1.2   Installation of R/Bioconductor Packages

Install the R/Bioconductor packages for miRNA microarray data analysis with `biocLite()`. The packages are summarized in Table 1 [5–16].

```
> biocLite(c("Biobase", "GEOquery", "limma", "mclust",
"devtools",
+ "GOstats","gplots","networkD3","miRNAtap","miRNAtap.db",
+ "visNetwork","SpidermiR"))
```

2.2   Datasets

A public available dataset, GSE54578, is used as an example for demonstration   (https://www.ncbi.nlm.nih.gov/geo/query/acc.cgi?acc=GSE54578). The study profiles genome-wide miRNA expression in blood from 15 early-onset schizophrenia cases and 15 healthy controls, detecting a total of 1070 miRNAs by the microarrays [17]. A GPL16016 platform (Exiqon miRCURY LNA microRNA array) was used [17]. The dataset can be downloaded through the link directly; alternatively, it can be accessed with "getGEO" function of the "GEOquery" package.

```
> library("GEOquery")
> gset <- getGEO("GSE54578",GSEMatrix=TRUE,AnnotGPL=FALSE)
```

Table 1
R packages used in the chapter for miRNA data analysis

Package name	Short description
Biobase [5]	Functions that are needed by many other packages or which replace R functions
devtools [6]	Collection of package development tools
GOstats [7]	Tools for manipulating GO and microarrays
GEOquery [8]	GEOquery is the bridge between GEO and BioConductor
gplots [9]	Various R programming tools for plotting data
limma [10]	Data analysis, linear models and differential expression for microarray data
mclust [11]	Gaussian finite mixture models fitted via EM algorithm for model-based clustering, classification, and density estimation
miRNAtap [12]	microRNA targets aggregated predictions
miRNAtap.db [13]	Holding the database for miRNAtap
networkD3 [14]	Creates 'D3' 'JavaScript' network, tree, dendrogram, and Sankey graphs from 'R'
SpidermiR [15]	The package provides multiple methods for query, prepare and download network data, and the integration with validated and predicted miRNA data and the use of standard analysis and visualization methods
visNetwork [16]	Provides an R interface to the 'vis.js' JavaScript charting library

```
> if(length(gset)>1) idx <- grep("GPL16016",attr(gset,"-
names")) else idx <- 1
> gset <- gset[[idx]]
```

The GSE54578 dataset is now stored in `gset`, which will be used for further processing and analysis.

3   Methods

3.1   Preprocessing and Normalization

3.1.1   Preprocessing

The original miRNA expression data could contain some "NA" values and the columns are named with GSM accessions in default. The data structure and content can be shown with "`head(exprs(gset))`" command (Fig. 1a). In the preprocessing step, we may wish to remove all the "NA" records and rename the columns with user-readable format (Fig. 1b).

```
> head(exprs(gset))
> rmv <- which(apply(exprs(gset),1,function(x) any (is.na
(x))))
```

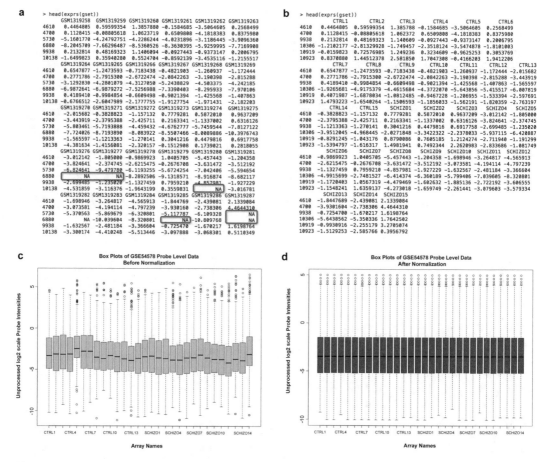

Fig. 1 Preprocessing of miRNA microarray data. (**a**) Raw expression data containing "NA" values. (**b**) "NA" filtered expression data. (**c**) Variance among samples before normalization. (**d**) Variance among samples after normalization

```
> gset <- gset[-rmv,]
> sampleNames(gset) <- c("CTRL1", ...,"CTRL15","SCHIZO1",...,"SCHIZO15")
> gsms <-"000000000000000111111111111111" #Grouping names
> sml <- c()
> for(i in 1:nchar(gsms)) {sml[i] <- substr(gsms,i,i)}
> head(exprs(gset))
```

Note that the "CTRL2"~"CTRL14" and "SCHI-ZO1"~"SCHIZO15" were omitted in the demonstrated command line.

Before normalization, the probe intensities should be checked to find out the apparent outliers caused by nonsystem errors. These outliers must be excluded for further analysis. Typically, a "box-plot" can be generated and show the uniformity of the signal intensity.

```
> ex <- exprs(gset)
> boxplot(ex, which='pm', ylab="Intensities", xlab="Array names")
```

After recalling and filtering the arrays with apparent experimental biases, the general signal intensity distribution should follow the distribution patterns as in Fig. 1c, with small variance among arrays.

3.1.2 Normalization

After preprocessing, the microarray data must be normalized to get rid of variations with nonbiological sources. A large number of methods have been proposed to normalize microarray-based transcriptome data. The methods are suited for different platforms and integrated in packages for corresponding data analysis, e.g., "NormiR" function in the "ExiMiR" package for two-color microarray experiments using a common reference or similar methods in the "affy" package for single-channel Affymetrix arrays, "normalizeBetweenArrays" function in the "limma" package, etc. In the example, "normalizeBetweenArrays" is applied, with a quantile normalization procedure.

```
> library("limma")
> ex_norm <- normalizeBetweenArrays(ex)
> qu <- as.numeric(quantile(ex,c(0.,0.25,0.5,0.75,0.99,1.0),
na.rm=T))
> filt <- ( qu[5]>100 || (qu[6]-qu[1]>50 && qu[2]>0) || (qu[2]>
0 && qu[2]<1 && qu[4]>1
&& qu[4]<2))
> if(filt){ex_norm[which(ex<=0)] <- NaN; exprs(gset) <- log2
(ex_norm)}
```

A log2 transformation is done to the normalized expression values to make the data follow Gaussian distribution more approximately. A boxplot generated with the normalized data shows more even distribution of the expression levels among different arrays (Fig. 1d).

3.2 Expression Difference and Clustering Analysis

The normalized expression data can be compared directly between groups. *T* Test is the most straightforward statistic comparison method between two groups, which will measure the significance of difference with probability of no difference (p values: the lower, the more significant). For microarray data, tens of thousands of genes are compared between groups simultaneously and it is a massive multiple testing problem. It is more complicated that the measured expression levels do not always follow normal distributions and have nonidentical and dependent distributions between genes. To solve this problem and identify the differentially expressed genes more precisely, Smyth proposed an empirical Bayes moderated t test, which has been incorporated into the "limma" package [10]. An example is shown as following, and more details about the usage of "eBayes" can refer to the document: http://web.mit.edu/~r/current/arch/i386_linux26/lib/R/library/limma/html/ebayes.html.

```
> sml <- paste("G",sml,sep="")
> fl <- as.factor(sml)
> gset$description <- fl
&gt; design &lt;- model.matrix(~ description + 0, gset)
> colnames(design) <- levels(fl)
> fit <- lmFit(gset,design)
> cont.matrix <- makeContrasts(G1-G0,levels=design)
> fit2 <- contrasts.fit(fit,cont.matrix)
> fit2 <- eBayes(fit2,0.01)
> tT <- topTable(fit2,adjust="fdr",sort.by="B",number=1000)
```

The comparison results are stored in objects *fit2* and *tT*, which will be used for further analysis.

Besides the significance measured by the statistic p values, the fold change amplitude of miRNA gene expression levels also appears important to biologists. A volcano plot can show the statistic significance and change amplitude in a two-dimensional plane simultaneously, which plots the fold change and p values (log-transformed results) on x- and y-axis respectively (Fig. 2a). The "volcanoplot" function in the "limma" package can be applied conveniently. Note that the 'highlight' argument indicates the top probe sets are highlighted. Other packages such as "ggplot2" also have functions to draw volcano plots.

```
> volcanoplot(fit2,coef=1,highlight=10)
```

Alternatively, basic R plot function can also generate the volcano plot.

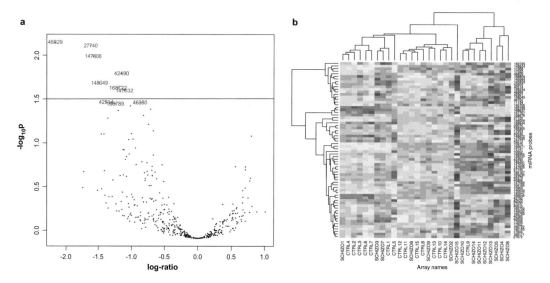

Fig. 2 Volcano plot and heat map of miRNA expression data. (**a**) Volcano plot showing the differentially expressed miRNAs between disease and control samples. (**b**) Clustering the samples and genes with expression patterns of significantly differential miRNAs

```
> lod <- -log10(tT$adj.P.Val)
> plot(tT$logFC,lod,xlab="log-ratio",ylab=expression(-log[10]~p))
> abline(h=1.5,col="red")
```

As in other transcriptome data analysis, besides gene expression difference analysis, clustering analysis can also be performed for miRNA microarray data. For example, a simple heatmap plot can be generated for a subset of the miRNAs with significant expression difference between disease and control (Fig. 2b; FDR adjusted p-value < 0.05).

```
> selected <- which(p.adjust(fit2$p.value[,1]<0.05) == 1)
> esetSel <- ex_norm[selected,]
> heatmap(esetSel)
```

For more in-depth clustering analysis, readers can refer to Chapter 2 of the book, since the procedure and tools are general rather than specific for miRNA datasets.

3.3 miRNA Target Analysis

The difference between miRNA and general transcriptome data analysis is mainly represented by the specific target gene analysis of the former. The major activity of miRNAs is to regulate the expression of target genes posttranscriptionally or translationally, and therefore annotation of the target genes of interesting miRNAs appears important.

3.3.1 Target Identification

There are multiple options to identify target genes of miRNAs. For example, Brock et al proposed a pipeline for miRNA target analysis with R packages "targetscan.Mm.eg.db", "micro-RNA" and "org.Mm.eg.db". In the example shown below, an integrated package "SpidermiR" is adopted, which provides both validated and predicted target genes from multiple databases or software tools including mirWalk [18], miR2Disease [19], miR-Tar [20], miRTarBase [21], miRandola [22], Pharmaco-miR [23], DIANA [24], Miranda [25], PicTar [26], and TargetScan [27]. It can also retrieve and visualize the gene networks. The following commands give an example of target gene determination for some interesting miRNAs, e.g., the top significant five miRNAs with expression difference between groups (*see* **Note 1**). The potential targets of these miRNAs will be predicted with SpidermiRdownload_miRNAprediction and exported to mirnaTar.

```
> tT[selected,]$Name[1:5]
> mirna <-
c('hsa-miR-4429','hsa-miR-1827','hsa-miR-5002-5p','hsa-miR-
5187-3p','hsa-miR-4455')
> mirnaTar <- SpidermiRdownload_miRNAprediction(mirna_list=-
mirna)
```

The data frame of `mirnaTar` can be checked with `head(mirnaTar)`, and there are two columns, `V1` showing miRNA names and `V2` listing the target genes.

Note that `SpidermiRdownload_miRNAprediction` gave the prediction targets of four tools: DIANA, Miranda, PicTar, and TargetScan. The validated targets could be downloaded from miRTAR and miRwalk with `SpidermiRdownload_miRNAvalidate` function.

3.3.2 Network and Gene Set Enrichment Analysis

Network analysis and visualization can show not only the shared targets of multiple miRNAs, but also the interactions and pathways among the target genes. There are many tools developed for network building and visualization, e.g., user-friendly interfaced tool Cytoscape [28], R package SpidermiR [15]. Here, we use Cytoscape to construct the regulatory network between the miRNAs (top significant 5) and their predicted targets (50 for each miRNA), since Cytoscape is quite straightforward and particularly useful for network construction with user-customized interactions (Fig. 3a) (*see* **Note 2**). GeneMANIA curates validated and predicted networks between genes from a variety of species [29]. The network types include coexpression, colocalization, genetic interactions, pathway, physical interactions, shared protein domains, and predicted interactions. GeneMANIA also provides a webserver to implement the network construction. SpidermiR can download the interaction data from GeneMANIA and visualize the networks among the user-customized genes, and the functions are still being debugged and updated. Here, we directly use the GeneMANIA prediction server (http://genemania.org/) to construct the pathway network of miRNA target genes (Fig. 3b) (*see* **Note 3**).

Besides the network analysis, statistics-based gene set enrichment analysis (GSEA) should be done for the miRNAs and miRNA targets, so as to find biological meanings and help increase the statistical power through aggregating the signal across groups of related genes. `GOstats` and a number of other R/Bioconductor packages (e.g., `GeneAnswers` [30]) can make the enrichment analysis with hypergeomtric tests (`hyperGTest` function for `GOstats`). As an example, we use `GOstats` to make GO enrichment analysis (Biological Process) to the predicted target genes of the top 5 miRNAs (*see* **Note 4**).

```
> library("org.Hs.eg.db")
> library("GSEABase")
> library("GOstats")
> mirTarget <- mirnaTar$V2
> goAnn <- get("org.Hs.egGO")
> universe <- Lkeys(goAnn)
> entrezIDs <- mget(mirTarget, org.Hs.egSYMBOL2EG, ifnotfound=NA)
> entrezIDs <- as.character(entrezIDs)
```

a

b

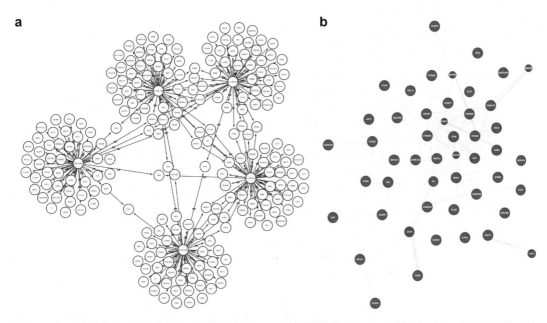

Fig. 3 Interaction networks among miRNAs and their targets. (**a**) Regulatory network between miRNAs and target genes. (**b**) Pathway sub-network among the miRNA target genes

```
> params <- new("GOHyperGParams",
+ geneIds=entrezIDs,
+ universeGeneIds=universe,
+ annotation="org.Hs.eg.db",
+ ontology="BP",
+ pvalueCutoff=0.01,
+ conditional=FALSE,
+ testDirection="over")
> goET <- hyperGTest(params)
> library(Category)
> genelist <- geneIdsByCategory(goET)
> genelist <- sapply(genelist, function(.ids) {
+ .sym &lt;- mget(.ids, envir=org.Hs.egSYMBOL, ifnotfound=NA)
+ .sym[is.na(.sym)] &lt;- .ids[is.na(.sym)]
+ paste(.sym, collapse=";")
+ })
> GObp <- summary(goET)
> GObp$Symbols <- genelist[as.character(GObp$GOBPID)]
> head(GObp)
```

KEGG enrichment can also be performed:

```
> keggAnn <- get("org.Hs.egPATH")
> universe <- Lkeys(keggAnn)
> params <- new("KEGGHyperGParams",
+ geneIds=entrezIDs,
```

```
+ universeGeneIds=universe,
+ annotation="org.Hs.eg.db",
+ categoryName="KEGG",
+ pvalueCutoff=0.01,
+ testDirection="over")
> keggET <- hyperGTest(params)
> kegg <- summary(keggET)
> library(Category)
> genelist <- geneIdsByCategory(keggET)
> genelist <- sapply(genelist, function(.ids) {
+ .sym <- mget(.ids, envir=org.Hs.egSYMBOL, ifnotfound=NA)
+ .sym[is.na(.sym)] <- .ids[is.na(.sym)]
+ paste(.sym, collapse=";")
+ })
> kegg$Symbols <- genelist[as.character(kegg$KEGGID)]
> head(kegg)
```

4 Notes

1. For illustration convenience, the top five miRNAs are selected
   for target analysis. In practice, all the meaningful miRNAs
   should be analyzed for targets. For target prediction, multiple
   prediction tools should be combined and the intersected set will
   be selected for further analysis if the number of prediction
   results is large.

2. Cytoscape can be downloaded from http://www.cytoscape.org.
   There is a detailed manual demonstrating how to install and use
   the tool. To visualize the interaction network of miRNAs and
   their target genes, a two-column table is prepared in which the
   first column records miRNAs and the second records the
   corresponding targets. Directly import the interaction table to
   Cytoscape, indicate the interaction sources and targets, and then
   draw the network with directions.

3. GeneMANIA curates several categories of gene interaction databases, and the database(s) can be selected in the server for
   network prediction. In the GeneMANIA prediction webserver
   (http://genemania.org), simply copy the gene symbols (one per
   line) into the input area, select the desired database(s) and run
   prediction.

4. Besides GOstats, there are also other R packages making Gene
   Set Enrichment Analysis (GSEA). Chapter 3 in this book can be
   referred to, which gives a comprehensive introduction on the
   methods and related packages. The website of Gene Ontology
   Consortium (http://geneontology.org) also presents an online
   GO enrichment analysis tool, and it would be an easy choice.

References

1. Kozomara A, Griffiths-Jones S (2014) miR-Base: annotating high confidence microRNAs using deep sequencing data. Nucleic Acids Res 42(Database issue):D68–D73. https://doi.org/10.1093/nar/gkt1181

2. McCall MN, Kim MS, Adil M, Patil AH, Lu Y, Mitchell CJ, Leal-Rojas P, Xu J, Kumar M, Dawson VL, Dawson TM, Baras AS, Rosenberg AZ, Arking DE, Burns KH, Pandey A, Halushka MK (2017) Toward the human cellular microRNAome. Genome Res. https://doi.org/10.1101/gr.222067.117

3. Otto T, Candido SV, Pilarz MS, Sicinska E, Bronson RT, Bowden M, Lachowicz IA, Mulry K, Fassl A, Han RC, Jecrois ES, Sicinski P (2017) Cell cycle-targeting microRNAs promote differentiation by enforcing cell-cycle exit. Proc Natl Acad Sci U S A 114 (40):10660–10665. pii 201702914. https://doi.org/10.1073/pnas.1702914114

4. Gao L, Jiang F (2016) MicroRNA (miRNA) profiling. Methods Mol Biol 1381:151–161

5. Huber W, Carey VJ, Gentleman R, Anders S, Carlson M, Carvalho BS, Bravo HC, Davis S, Gatto L, Girke T, Gottardo R, Hahne F, Hansen KD, Irizarry RA, Lawrence M, Love MI, MacDonald J, Obenchain V, Oleś AK, Pagès H, Reyes A, Shannon P, Smyth GK, Tenenbaum D, Waldron L, Morgan M (2015) Orchestrating high-throughput genomic analysis with Bioconductor. Nat Methods 12(2):115–121. https://doi.org/10.1038/nmeth.3252

6. Wickham H, Chang W (2017) devtools: tools to make developing R packages easier. R package version 1.13.3. https://CRAN.R-project.org/package=devtools.

7. Falcon S, Gentleman R (2007) Using GOstats to test gene lists for GO term association. Bioinformatics 23(2):257–258

8. Davis S, Meltzer PS (2017) GEOquery: a bridge between the Gene Expression Omnibus (GEO) and BioConductor. Bioinformatics 23 (14):1846–1847

9. Warnes GR, Bolker B, Bonebakker L, et al. (2016) gplots: various R programming tools for plotting data. R package version 3.0.1. https://CRAN.R-project.org/package=gplots.

10. Ritchie ME, Phipson B, Wu D, Hu Y, Law CW, Shi W, Smyth GK (2015) limma powers differential expression analyses for RNA-sequencing and microarray studies. Nucleic Acids Res 43 (7):e47

11. Scrucca L, Fop M, Murphy TB, Raftery AE (2016) mclust 5: clustering, classification and density estimation using Gaussian finite mixture models. R J 8(1):289–317

12. Pajak M, Simpson TI (2016) miRNAtap: miRNAtap: microRNA targets – aggregated predictions. R package version 1.8.0.

13. Pajak M, Simpson TI (2016) miRNAtap.db: data for miRNAtap. R package version 0.99.10.

14. Allaire JJ, Gandrud C, Russell K, Yetman CJ (2017) networkD3: D3 JavaScript network graphs from R. R package version 0.4. https://CRAN.R-project.org/package=networkD3.

15. Cava C, Colaprico A, Bertoli G, Graudenzi A, Silva TC, Olsen C, Noushmehr H, Bontempi G, Mauri G, Castiglioni I (2017) SpidermiR: an R/bioconductor package for integrative analysis with miRNA data. Int J Mol Sci 18(2.): pii: E274). https://doi.org/10.3390/ijms18020274

16. Almende BV, Thieurmel B, Robert T (2017) visNetwork: network visualization using 'vis.js' library. R package version 2.0.1. https://CRAN.R-project.org/package=visNetwork.

17. Zhang F, Xu Y, Shugart YY, Yue W et al (2015) Converging evidence implicates the abnormal microRNA system in schizophrenia. Schizophr Bull 41(3):728–735

18. Dweep H, Sticht C, Pandey P, Gretz N (2011) miRWalk--database: prediction of possible miRNA binding sites by "walking" the genes of three genomes. J Biomed Inform 44 (5):839–847

19. Jiang Q, Wang Y, Hao Y, Juan L, Teng M, Zhang X, Li M, Wang G, Liu Y (2009) miR2Disease: a manually curated database for microRNA deregulation in human disease. Nucleic Acids Res 37(Database issue):D98–104

20. Hsu JB, Chiu CM, Hsu SD, Huang WY, Chien CH, Lee TY, Huang HD (2011) miRTar: an integrated system for identifying miRNA-target interactions in human. BMC Bioinformatics 12:300. https://doi.org/10.1186/1471-2105-12-300

21. Hsu SD, Lin FM, Wu WY, Liang C, Huang WC, Chan WL, Tsai WT, Chen GZ, Lee CJ, Chiu CM, Chien CH, Wu MC, Huang CY, Tsou AP, Huang HD (2011) miRTarBase: a database curates experimentally validated microRNA-target interactions. Nucleic Acids Res 39(Database issue):D163–D169. https://doi.org/10.1093/nar/gkq1107

22. Russo F, Di Bella S, Nigita G, Macca V, Laganà A, Giugno R, Pulvirenti A, Ferro A (2012) miRandola: extracellular circulating microRNAs database. PLoS One 7(10):e47786. https://doi.org/10.1371/journal.pone.0047786

23. Rukov JL, Wilentzik R, Jaffe I, Vinther J, Shomron N (2014) Pharmaco-miR: linking microRNAs and drug effects. Brief Bioinform 15(4):648–659. https://doi.org/10.1093/bib/bbs082

24. Maragkakis M, Reczko M, Simossis VA, Alexiou P, Papadopoulos GL, Dalamagas T, Giannopoulos G, Goumas G, Koukis E, Kourtis K, Vergoulis T, Koziris N, Sellis T, Tsanakas P, Hatzigeorgiou AG (2009) DIANA-microT web server: elucidating microRNA functions through target prediction. Nucleic Acids Res 37(Web Server issue):W273–W276

25. John B, Enright AJ, Aravin A, Tuschl T, Sander C, Marks DS (2004) Human MicroRNA targets. PLoS Biol 2(11):e363

26. Krek A, Grün D, Poy MN, Wolf R, Rosenberg L, Epstein EJ, MacMenamin P, da Piedade I, Gunsalus KC, Stoffel M, Rajewsky N (2005) Combinatorial microRNA target predictions. Nat Genet 37(5):495–500

27. Agarwal V, Bell GW, Nam J, Bartel DP (2015) Predicting effective microRNA target sites in mammalian mRNAs. eLife 4:e05005

28. Saito R, Smoot ME, Ono K, Ruscheinski J, Wang PL, Lotia S, Pico AR, Bader GD, Ideker T (2012) A travel guide to cytoscape plugins. Nat Methods 9(11):1069–1076. https://doi.org/10.1038/nmeth.2212

29. Montojo J, Zuberi K, Rodriguez H, Bader GD, Morris Q (2014) GeneMANIA: fast gene network construction and function prediction for cytoscape. F1000Res 3(153). https://doi.org/10.12688/f1000research.4572.1. eCollection 2014

30. Feng G, Shaw P, Rosen ST, Lin SM, Kibbe WA (2012) Using the bioconductor GeneAnswers package to interpret gene lists. Methods Mol Biol 802:101–112. https://doi.org/10.1007/978-1-61779-400-1_7

Chapter 10

Identification and Expression Analysis of Long Intergenic Noncoding RNAs

Ming-an Sun, Rihong Zhai, Qing Zhang, and Yejun Wang

Abstract

Long intergenic noncoding RNAs (lincRNAs) have caught increasing attention in recent years. The advance of RNA-Seq has greatly facilitated the discovery of novel lincRNAs. However, the computational analysis of lincRNAs is still challenging. In this protocol, we presented a step-by-step protocol for computational analyses of lincRNAs, including read processing and alignment, transcript assembly, lincRNA identification and annotation, and differential expression analysis.

Key words Noncoding RNA, lncRNA, lincRNA, RNA-Seq, Differential expression, STAR, Cufflinks, CPAT

1 Introduction

The sequencing of human genome [1] identified approximately 20,000–25,000 protein coding genes, which represent less than 2% of the whole genome. Later studies suggested that transcription is not limited to protein-coding regions, and more than 90% of the human genome is likely to be transcribed [2], which produces a variety of noncoding RNAs [3–5], including microRNAs, piwi-interacting RNAs, circular RNAs, and long noncoding RNAs.

GENCODE v7 [6] divided long noncoding RNAs (lncRNAs) into 12 biotypes based on their genetic markup and potential function. Among them, long intergenic noncoding RNAs (lincRNAs), which are noncoding RNAs longer than 200 bp transcribed from the intergenic regions of protein coding genes, have caught increasing attentions in recent years [3]. While the function of most lincRNAs remains to be explored, many of them seem to be functionally important given that they typically show distinct tissue and cell-type specific expression [7, 8], and are associated with different tumors and diseases [9, 10]. Recent work suggested that lincRNAs are involved in various layers of regulation, including chromatin

Yejun Wang and Ming-an Sun (eds.), *Transcriptome Data Analysis: Methods and Protocols*, Methods in Molecular Biology, vol. 1751, https://doi.org/10.1007/978-1-4939-7710-9_10, © Springer Science+Business Media, LLC 2018

programming, cis regulation at enhancers, and posttranscriptional regulation of mRNA processing [11, 12].

The emergence of high-throughput RNA-Seq has greatly facilitated the systematic identification of lincRNAs [7, 13]. Recently, single-cell RNA-Seq has also been adopted to investigate the cell-specific expression of lincRNA and other noncoding RNAs [14]. The most recent release of NONCODE database has collected >30,000 human lincRNAs [15]. Meanwhile, lincRNAs are also increasingly studied in other model and non-model species. Comparison among different species indicated that lincRNAs are less conserved than protein-coding genes [6].

In this protocol, we presented a step-by-step protocol for computational analyses of lincRNAs, including RNA-Seq read processing and alignment, transcript assembly, lincRNA identification and annotation, and differential expression analysis.

2   Materials

2.1 Hardware and Software Requirement

Most of the tools used in this protocol are developed for Linux Operating System (e.g., Ubuntu, RedHat, CentoOS, and Federa), thus a computer with Linux environment is required. All the steps described in this protocol have been tested on a high-performance computer (56 CPU, 252 Gb memory) with 64-bit CentOS (release 6.8) installed. All tools involved are summarized in Table 1. To be

Table 1
Bioinformatic tools used in this protocol

Software	Function	URL
Sratoolkit (v2.8.1)	Extract FastQ files from SRA database	https://www.ncbi.nlm.nih.gov/sra/docs/toolkitsoft
FastQC (v0.11.5)	Quality control for high-throughput sequencing data	https://www.bioinformatics.babraham.ac.uk/projects/fastqc
Trim Galore (v0.4.2)	Read processing, including adaptor removal and bad quality base trimming	https://www.bioinformatics.babraham.ac.uk/projects/trim_galore
Cutadapt (v1.12)	Invoked by Trim Galore for read processing	http://cutadapt.readthedocs.io/en/stable/index.html
STAR (v.2.5.3)	Read alignment	https://github.com/alexdobin/STAR
Samtools (v1.4)	BAM/SAM/CRAM file reading, writing, editing, indexing, and viewing	https://github.com/samtools/samtools
Cufflinks (v2.2.1)	Transcript assembly, quantification, and differential analysis	https://github.com/cole-trapnell-lab/cufflinks
CPAT (v1.2.2)	Coding potential assessment	http://rna-cpat.sourceforge.net

noted, even though most of the tools can be used under modern PC, large amount of memory (around 30 Gb for mammalian genome) is necessary to run STAR [16] (*see* **Note 1**).

2.2 RNA-Seq Data

This protocol starts with FastQ files for RNA-Seq datasets. Most publicly available RNA-Seq datasets could be obtained from NCBI Gene Expression Omnibus (GEO; https://www.ncbi.nlm.nih.gov/geo/). For demonstration, here we used two RNA-Seq datasets from ENCODE project—for mouse embryonic day 14.5 (*E*.14.5) brain (GEO accession: GSE90197) and liver (GEO accession: GSE90196), respectively. Both are paired-end data with two biological replicates, sequenced from stranded rRNA-depleted Poly-A+ RNA-Seq libraries of longer than 200 nucleotides in size.

2.3 Annotation Files

In this protocol, two types of annotation files are required: (1) reference genome sequences of FASTA format; (2) gene annotation file of GTF format, which includes both protein coding and noncoding genes. These files can usually be obtained from databases like UCSC Genome Browser, Ensembl or GENCODE. Here, we downloaded mouse reference genome and gene annotation file of Release M14 (GRCm38.p5) from GENCODE [6]: https://www.gencodegenes.org/mouse_releases/current.html. These files can be downloaded with Linux command *wget* and uncompressed for use:

```
# download
wget ftp://ftp.sanger.ac.uk/pub/gencode/Gencode_mouse/relea-
se_M14/GRCm38.p5.genome.fa.gz
wget ftp://ftp.sanger.ac.uk/pub/gencode/Gencode_mouse/relea-
se_M14/gencode.vM14.annotation.gtf.gz
# uncompress the downloaded files
gunzip GRCm38.p5.genome.fa.gz
gunzip gencode.vM14.annotation.gtf.gz
```

3 Methods

3.1 Data Preparation

1. Sratoolkit installation. The precompiled executes of sratoolkits [17] for different platforms can be downloaded for use. To get its 64-bit version for CentOS, type:

```
# download
wget
http://ftp-trace.ncbi.nlm.nih.gov/sra/sdk/current/
sratoolkit.current-centos_linux64.tar.gz
# uncompress
tar xvf sratoolkit.current-centos_linux64.tar.gz
# add execute directory to PATH
export PATH=$PATH:/path/to/sratoolkit.2.8.2-1-centos_
linux64/bin
```

2. We obtained the RNA-Seq data from GEO (https://www.ncbi.nlm.nih.gov/geo/) by searching GEO accession. Follow the links to specific samples and then SRA database, you can find detailed information including the SRA accession number. For example, the SRA accession for the brain sample replicate 1 is SRR5048019. The FastQ files of this dataset can be generated by using the *fastq-dump* command from sra-toolkits (*see* **Note 2**). In the terminal, type:

```
fastq-dump --split-3 SRR5048019
```

3. After the command is finished, FastQ files for read 1 and 2 (e.g., SRR5048019_1.fastq and SRR5048019_2.fastq for this case) respectively will be generated in the working directory. To simplify following analysis, the FastQ files are renamed to easier names (i.e., brain_rep1_1.fastq, brain_rep1_2.fastq, etc.), using the *mv* command:

```
mv SRR5048019_1.fastq brain_rep1_1.fastq
mv SRR5048019_2.fastq brain_rep1_2.fastq
```

3.2 Quality Control

1. FastQC installation. For quality assessment of the data, we used FastQC [18] which is a convenient tool for quality controlling on high throughput sequencing data. It can be downloaded from https://www.bioinformatics.babraham.ac.uk/projects/fastqc/. It can be used on a computer with JRE installed.

2. To get quality assessment of a FastQ file (e.g., brain_rep1_1.fastq), simply type (*see* **Note 3**):

```
fastqc brain_rep1_1.fastq
```

The quality assessment results will be saved as html files (e.g., brain_rep1_1.html) which show a variety of statistics for sequencing quality, adaptor occurrence, etc. (Figure 1).

3.3 Adaptor Removal and Read Trimming

1. *Trim Galore installation.* Trim Galore [19] is a tool to automate quality and adapter trimming. It can be downloaded from https://www.bioinformatics.babraham.ac.uk/projects/trim_galore/. It invokes Cutadapt [20] for adapter removal and bad quality bases trimming, thus Cutadapt needs to be installed in advance. Compared with Cutadapt, Trim Galore provides additional user-friendly functions (such as automatic determination of the overrepresented adaptors).

```
# download
wget https://github.com/FelixKrueger/TrimGalore/archive/
0.4.2.tar.gz
# uncompress, which will generate a folder named TrimGalore-
0.4.2 in this case
tar xvzf 0.4.2.tar.gz
# export execute folder to PATH
export PATH=$PATH:/path/to/TrimGalore-0.4.2
```

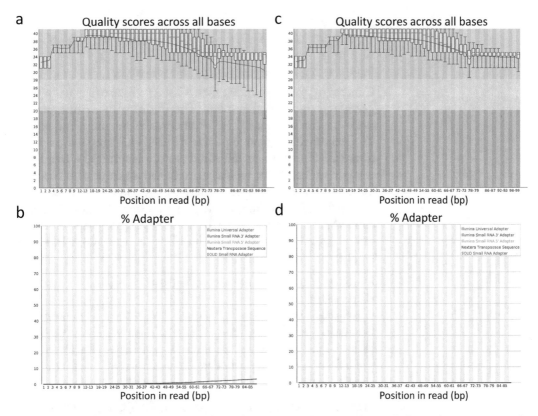

Fig. 1 Quality control report generated by FastQC before and after trimming. (**a, b**) Per-base sequence quality and adapter content before trimming. (**c, d**) Per-base sequence quality and adapter content after trimming by Trim Galore. The data for SRR5048019_1.fastq is used for demonstration

2. To preprocess a pair of FastQ files (e.g., brain_rep1_1.fastq and brain_rep1_2.fastq), type:

```
trim_galore --phred33 --illumina --paired --length
20 brain_rep1_1.fastq brain_rep1_2.fastq
```

Trimmed FastQ files with names like brain_rep1_1_val_1.fastq and brain_rep1_2_val_2.fastq will be generated for read 1 and read 2, respectively.

3. Rerun FastQC after read trimming. As shown in Fig. 1c, d, bad quality bases and sequencing adaptors are removed after this step.

3.4 Read Alignment to Reference Genome

1. STAR installation. In this protocol, we used STAR [16] to align reads to the reference genome. The source codes can be downloaded from its web site, and then uncompressed and compiled by typing:

```
# download source code
wget https://github.com/alexdobin/STAR/archive/2.5.3a.tar.gz
# uncompress the tar ball, and go to the source directory
tar -xzvf 2.5.3a.tar.gz
```

```
cd STAR-2.5.3a
# build STAR, and export the execute directory to PATH
make STAR
export PATH=/directory/to/STAR-2.5.3a:$PATH
```

2. Generating genome index files. Genome index files need to be generated for read alignment. The folder with writing permissions has to be created in advance to store these index files. The reference genome sequences (FASTA file) and gene annotations (GTF file) are needed. In this step, around 30 Gb of memory is required for a typical mammalian genome (*see* **Note 1**). Take the aforementioned reference genome sequences (i.e., GRCm38.p5.genome.fa) and gene annotation files (i.e., gencode.vM14.annotation.gtf) for mouse as example, the index files can be generated to a specified folder (i.e., mm10StarIndex) by typing:

```
# create a folder named mm10StarIndex
mkdir mm10StarIndex
# Generate STAR index files to the folder mm10StarIndex.
Parameter -runThreadN specifies the number of CPU to use.
STAR --runMode genomeGenerate --genomeDir mm10StarIndex
--genomeFastaFiles GRCm38.p5.genome.fa --sjdbGTFfile
gencode.vM14.annotation.gtf --runThreadN 8
```

3. Mapping reads to reference genome. STAR maps the reads to the genome, and writes several output files, such as alignments (SAM/BAM), mapping summary statistics, splice junctions, unmapped reads, signal (wiggle) tracks etc. To map paired-end reads of brain samples (i.e., brain_rep1_1_val_1.fastq brain_rep1_2_val_2.fastq) to mouse genome, type:

```
STAR --runThreadN 12 --genomeDir mm10StarIndex --genomeLoad
LoadAndRemove --readFilesIn brain_rep1_1_val_1.fastq
brain_rep1_2_val_2.fastq --outSAMtype BAM Unsorted -outStd
SAM --outSAMattributes Standard --outSAMunmapped None --
outFilterType BySJout --outFilterMismatchNmax 10
--outFileNamePrefix brain_rep1.
```

After mapping, BAM files with suffix ".Aligned.out.bam", along with several log files with basic statistics will be generated.

4. Samtools installation. The generated BAM files should be sorted by position or read names for following analysis. Samtools [21] provide a collection of tools for handling BAM/SAM/CRAM files, including sorting. Take the version 1.4 for example, it can be installed by:

```
# download source code
wget
```

```
https://github.com/samtools/samtools/releases/download/
1.4/samtools-1.4.tar.bz2
# uncompress the tar ball, and go to the folder
tar xvf samtools-1.4.tar.gz2
cd samtools-1.4
# configure and install
./configure --prefix=/path/to/install
make
make install
# export the execute directory to PATH
export PATH=$PATH:/path/to/install/bin
```

5. Sorting BAM files. The *sort* function from samtools can be used to sort BAM files, either by position or read name. Take brain_rep1.Aligned.out.bam as example, to sort it by position and save as brain_rep1.srt.bam, type:

```
samtools sort -o brain_rep1.srt.bam brain_rep1.Aligned.out.bam
```

The parameters -o sets the name of the sorted BAM file to be generated. Alternatively, if the BAM file needs to be sorted by read name, the -n parameter needs to be specified. Type:

```
samtools sort -n -o brain_rep1.srt.bam brain_rep1.Aligned.out.
bam
```

3.5 Transcriptome Assembly

The Cufflinks package [22] provides a collection of programs for transcripts assembly, quantification and differential expression analysis.

1. Cufflinks installation. The precompiled binary release of cufflinks for several platforms can be downloaded for use after uncompression. Take v2.2.1 for 64-bit Linux as example, it can be obtained by:

```
# download the tar ball
wget
http://cole-trapnell-lab.github.io/cufflinks/assets/
downloads/cufflinks-2.2.1.Linux_x86_64.tar.gz
# uncompress, and export execute directory to PATH
tar -xzvf cufflinks-2.2.1.Linux_x86_64.tar.gz
export PATH=$PATH:/path/to/cufflinks-2.2.1.Linux_x86_64/
```

2. Transcript assembly. Transcript assembly can be conducted by the *cufflinks* function from Cufflinks package. If the users focus only on known transcripts in the provided GTF file, supply the GTF file (i.e., gencode.vM14.annotation.gtf) by parameter –G (*see* **Note 4**):

```
cufflinks -o brain_rep1.clgout -p 12 -G ./gencode.vM14.annota-
tion.gtf --library-type fr-firststrand brain_rep1.srt.bam
```

The parameters -o specifies output folder, -p specifies number of CPU for use, --library-type specifies library type for the RNA-Seq (*see* **Note 5**). In the output folder, information for all assembled transcripts is saved as transcripts.gtf.

3. Assembly merging. The assembly produced for each sample can be merged with the *cuffmerge* function from Cufflinks package. By supplying GTF file for known gene transcripts, novel transcripts identified from each sample together with known ones will be merged into a single GTF file. Take the GTF files from the four samples as example, first make a file with the path for all transcripts.gtf files:

```
ls */transcripts.gtf >assemblies.txt
```

Then run *cuffmerge*, with the result outputted to the folder cuffmerge_out:

```
cuffmerge -o cuffmerge_out -p 12 assemblies.txt
```

The file merged.gtf in the output folder contains the information for all assembled transcripts.

3.6 Identification of lincRNAs

The assembled transcripts include not only noncoding but also protein-coding genes. Thus it needs to be further screened for lincRNAs based on several criteria, including their length, genomic distribution and coding potential. Below we show how to screen for potential lincRNAs by several steps.

1. Installation of CPAT. CPAT [23] is a popular tool to evaluate coding potential (*see* **Note 6**). Both the standalone and online version of CPAT are available from: http://lilab.research.bcm.edu/cpat/. To download and install the standalone version (*see* **Note 7**), type:

```
# download source code and uncompress
wget https://sourceforge.net/projects/rna-cpat/files/
v1.2.2/CPAT-1.2.2.tar.gz
tar xzvf CPAT-1.2.2.tar.gz
# change working directory
cd CPAT-1.2.2
# build, install and export execute directory to PATH
python setup.py build
python setup.py install
export PATH=$PATH:/path/to/CPAT-1.2.2/bin
```

2. Transcript sequence extraction. Using the *gtfread* script from Cufflinks, the transcript sequences can be extracted based on the GTF file and reference genome sequences. The parameter -g specifies the FASTA file for reference genome, and -w for the FASTA file for the transcripts sequences to be generated.

```
gffread cuffmerge_out/merged.gtf -g ./GRCm38.p5.genome.fa -
w merged.fa
```

3. Evaluation of coding potential. The main script for CPAT is *cpat. py*, which can be used to evaluate the coding potential. Several parameters need to be specified, including -g for gene file (either in BED format or mRNA sequences), -o for output file, -x for prebuilt hexamer frequency table, -d for prebuilt training mode, and several other parameters. The prebuilt model files for several model organisms including human, mouse etc can be found in the dat subfolder of the installation directory. Otherwise, these files can be generated by using *make_hexamer_tab.py* and *make_- logitModel.py*, respectively. To apply CPAT to the file merged.fa generated last step, type:

```
cpat.py -g merged.fa -x ./ CPAT-1.2.2/dat/Mouse_Hexamer.tsv
-d ./CPAT-1.2.2/dat/Mouse_logitModel.RData -o merged.cpat.txt
```

The output file merged.cpat.txt is a tab separated file with each column as geneID, mRNA size, ORF size, Fickett Score, Hexamer Score, and Coding Probability (Table 2). By further applying a cutoff to the predicted coding probability, each transcript can be classified as protein coding or noncoding. The optimal cut-off for several model organisms can be found in the dat subfolder of the installation directory. For mouse, the cutoff is 0.44 as shown in Mouse_cutoff.txt. For species without pre-determined cut-off, the optimal cut-off can be estimated with known protein-coding and non-coding transcripts by cross-valication.

Table 2
Example lines of coding potential result predicted by CPAT

Sequence name	RNA size	ORF size	Ficket score	Hexamer score	Coding probability
CUFF.102562.1	648	69	0.5311	−0.83254	0.000763704
CUFF.102563.1	348	84	1.0898	−0.26818	0.023778568
CUFF.102565.1	942	72	0.9085	−1.07551	0.000579187
CUFF.102564.1	566	27	0.5386	−0.33633	0.004342168
CUFF.102566.1	559	237	0.495	0.184973	0.133638259
CUFF.102561.1	5953	612	1.2804	0.555167	0.975519766
CUFF.102561.2	6179	600	1.233	0.528778	0.967616482
CUFF.102567.1	572	288	0.8412	−0.56707	0.019221271
CUFF.102534.1	3619	174	0.5527	−0.49295	0.006307512
CUFF.102562.1	648	69	0.5311	−0.83254	0.000763704
CUFF.102563.1	348	84	1.0898	−0.26818	0.023778568

4. Screen against known protein domains. To remove transcripts that have similarity to known protein domains, first translate the nucleotide sequences for transcripts in all three sense frames use online tools or custom scripts, and then searched against Pfam database [24] at http://pfam.xfam.org. Alternatively, the users can search the nucleotide sequence against Pfam using the *hmmscan* function of HMMER. Any transcripts with significant similarity to Pfam protein domains are considered as protein-coding and discarded.

5. Filtering by length and genomic distribution. The putative non-coding RNAs obtained in last step are further screened for length. Those longer than 200 bp are considered as long noncoding RNAs (lncRNAs). To be noted, many studies also exclude mono-exonic transcripts to reduce the possibility of false positive discovery. By crossing against known genes, lncRNAs without any overlap with other protein coding genes are classified as lincRNAs.

3.7 Differential Expression Analysis

One of the major purposes of transcriptome analysis is to detect differentially expressed genes between different conditions (e.g., normal vs. tumor, treatment vs. untreatment). Differential expression analysis can be performed using the *cuffdiff* function from Cufflinks package (*see* **Note 8**). Cuffdiff takes the GTF file generated by *cuffmerge* and the sorted BAM files as input. Additional parameters also need to be specified, such as -L for condition labels, -p for numbers of CPU for use, --library-type for library type and -o for output dir. For example, to identify differential genes between brain and liver, type:

```
cuffdiff merged.gtf brain_rep1.srt.bam,brain_rep2.srt.bam
liver_rep1.srt.bam,liver_rep2.srt.bam -L brain,liver -p
8 --library-type fr-firststrand -o cuffdiff_out
```

In the cuffdiff_out folder, gene_exp.diff is the result for gene-level differential expression, and isoform_exp.diff is the result for transcript-level differential expression. These files include information such as gene/transcript information, expression in each sample, log2(fold_change), p-value, and q-value. The users can further filter the differential analysis results based on the lincRNA list obtained in last step for further analysis.

4   Notes

1. STAR outperforms most other aligners by a factor of >50 in mapping speed [16], however it requires large amount of memory. If no high-performance computer is available, the researchers can consider to use alternative mapping tools such as Tophat [25], which is more memory efficient and can run in most modern PC.

2. By providing the SRA accession number to *fastq-dump*, it can download sra files automatically and then generate FastQ files. Alternatively, the users can first download sra files from SRA database, then provide the sra file name to *fastq-dump* to generate FastQ files. The parameter --split-3 enables the splitting for mate-pairs, with read1 and read2 from paired-end sequencing placed in files *_1.fastq and *_2.fastq. For single-ended sequencing data, all reads will be placed in the file *.fastq.

3. To run FastQC, Java Run Environment is required. It can be downloaded from http://www.oracle.com/technetwork/java/javase/downloads/index.html. FastQC also provides a nice GUI interface which is user friendly for researchers unfamiliar with Linux terminal.

4. Alternatively, by specifying -g parameter, the users can apply a reference annotation based transcript (RABT) assembly method [26] to identify novel transcripts from RNA-Seq data.

5. Cufflinks support different types of RNA-Seq libraries, including ff-firststrand, ff-secondstrand, ff-unstranded, fr-firststrand, fr-secondstrand, fr-unstranded, and transfrags. The users need to make sure that the correct one is selected.

6. There are several alternative approaches for assessing transcript coding potential, such as CPC [27]. Multiple approaches can be used in combination to increase the realiability of the prediction.

7. R statistical language is required for CPAT to run properly. The users can download and install R based on instructions from: https://www.r-project.org/.

8. If the users are only interested in the differential expression at gene level, the users can choose to use count-based tools like DESeq2 [28] or edgeR [29] to identify differentially expressed genes.

Acknowledgments

This work was supported by a Natural Science Funding of Shenzhen (JCYJ201607115221141) and a Shenzhen Peacock Plan fund (827-000116) to Y.W. The funders had no role in study design, data collection and analysis, decision to publish, or preparation of the manuscript.

References

1. International Human Genome Sequencing C (2004) Finishing the euchromatic sequence of the human genome. Nature 431 (7011):931–945. https://doi.org/10.1038/nature03001

2. Consortium EP, Birney E, Stamatoyannopoulos JA, Dutta A, Guigo R, Gingeras TR, Margulies EH, Weng Z, Snyder M, Dermitzakis ET, Thurman RE, Kuehn MS, Taylor CM, Neph S, Koch CM, Asthana S, Malhotra A,

Adzhubei I, Greenbaum JA, Andrews RM, Flicek P, Boyle PJ, Cao H, Carter NP, Clelland GK, Davis S, Day N, Dhami P, Dillon SC, Dorschner MO, Fiegler H, Giresi PG, Goldy J, Hawrylycz M, Haydock A, Humbert R, James KD, Johnson BE, Johnson EM, Frum TT, Rosenzweig ER, Karnani N, Lee K, Lefebvre GC, Navas PA, Neri F, Parker SC, Sabo PJ, Sandstrom R, Shafer A, Vetrie D, Weaver M, Wilcox S, Yu M, Collins FS, Dekker J, Lieb JD, Tullius TD, Crawford GE, Sunyaev S, Noble WS, Dunham I, Denoeud F, Reymond A, Kapranov P, Rozowsky J, Zheng D, Castelo R, Frankish A, Harrow J, Ghosh S, Sandelin A, Hofacker IL, Baertsch R, Keefe D, Dike S, Cheng J, Hirsch HA, Sekinger EA, Lagarde J, Abril JF, Shahab A, Flamm C, Fried C, Hackermuller J, Hertel J, Lindemeyer M, Missal K, Tanzer A, Washietl S, Korbel J, Emanuelsson O, Pedersen JS, Holroyd N, Taylor R, Swarbreck D, Matthews N, Dickson MC, Thomas DJ, Weirauch MT, Gilbert J, Drenkow J, Bell I, Zhao X, Srinivasan KG, Sung WK, Ooi HS, Chiu KP, Foissac S, Alioto T, Brent M, Pachter L, Tress ML, Valencia A, Choo SW, Choo CY, Ucla C, Manzano C, Wyss C, Cheung E, Clark TG, Brown JB, Ganesh M, Patel S, Tammana H, Chrast J, Henrichsen CN, Kai C, Kawai J, Nagalakshmi U, Wu J, Lian Z, Lian J, Newburger P, Zhang X, Bickel P, Mattick JS, Carninci P, Hayashizaki Y, Weissman S, Hubbard T, Myers RM, Rogers J, Stadler PF, Lowe TM, Wei CL, Ruan Y, Struhl K, Gerstein M, Antonarakis SE, Fu Y, Green ED, Karaoz U, Siepel A, Taylor J, Liefer LA, Wetterstrand KA, Good PJ, Feingold EA, Guyer MS, Cooper GM, Asimenos G, Dewey CN, Hou M, Nikolaev S, Montoya-Burgos JI, Loytynoja A, Whelan S, Pardi F, Massingham T, Huang H, Zhang NR, Holmes I, Mullikin JC, Ureta-Vidal A, Paten B, Seringhaus M, Church D, Rosenbloom K, Kent WJ, Stone EA, Program NCS, Baylor College of Medicine Human Genome Sequencing C, Washington University Genome Sequencing C, Broad I, Children's Hospital Oakland Research I, Batzoglou S, Goldman N, Hardison RC, Haussler D, Miller W, Sidow A, Trinklein ND, Zhang ZD, Barrera L, Stuart R, King DC, Ameur A, Enroth S, Bieda MC, Kim J, Bhinge AA, Jiang N, Liu J, Yao F, Vega VB, Lee CW, Ng P, Shahab A, Yang A, Moqtaderi Z, Zhu Z, Xu X, Squazzo S, Oberley MJ, Inman D, Singer MA, Richmond TA, Munn KJ, Rada-Iglesias A, Wallerman O, Komorowski J, Fowler JC, Couttet P, Bruce AW, Dovey OM, Ellis PD, Langford CF, Nix DA, Euskirchen G, Hartman S, Urban AE, Kraus P, Van Calcar S, Heintzman N, Kim TH, Wang K, Qu C, Hon G, Luna R, Glass CK, Rosenfeld MG, Aldred SF, Cooper SJ, Halees A, Lin JM, Shulha HP, Zhang X, Xu M, Haidar JN, Yu Y, Ruan Y, Iyer VR, Green RD, Wadelius C, Farnham PJ, Ren B, Harte RA, Hinrichs AS, Trumbower H, Clawson H, Hillman-Jackson J, Zweig AS, Smith K, Thakkapallayil A, Barber G, Kuhn RM, Karolchik D, Armengol L, Bird CP, de Bakker PI, Kern AD, Lopez-Bigas N, Martin JD, Stranger BE, Woodroffe A, Davydov E, Dimas A, Eyras E, Hallgrimsdottir IB, Huppert J, Zody MC, Abecasis GR, Estivill X, Bouffard GG, Guan X, Hansen NF, Idol JR, Maduro VV, Maskeri B, McDowell JC, Park M, Thomas PJ, Young AC, Blakesley RW, Muzny DM, Sodergren E, Wheeler DA, Worley KC, Jiang H, Weinstock GM, Gibbs RA, Graves T, Fulton R, Mardis ER, Wilson RK, Clamp M, Cuff J, Gnerre S, Jaffe DB, Chang JL, Lindblad-Toh K, Lander ES, Koriabine M, Nefedov M, Osoegawa K, Yoshinaga Y, Zhu B, de Jong PJ (2007) Identification and analysis of functional elements in 1% of the human genome by the ENCODE pilot project. Nature 447(7146):799–816. https://doi.org/10.1038/nature05874

3. Mercer TR, Dinger ME, Mattick JS (2009) Long non-coding RNAs: insights into functions. Nat Rev Genet 10(3):155–159. https://doi.org/10.1038/nrg2521

4. Wilusz JE, Sunwoo H, Spector DL (2009) Long noncoding RNAs: functional surprises from the RNA world. Genes Dev 23 (13):1494–1504. https://doi.org/10.1101/gad.1800909

5. Bahn JH, Zhang Q, Li F, Chan TM, Lin X, Kim Y, Wong DT, Xiao X (2015) The landscape of microRNA, Piwi-interacting RNA, and circular RNA in human saliva. Clin Chem 61(1):221–230. https://doi.org/10.1373/clinchem.2014.230433

6. Derrien T, Johnson R, Bussotti G, Tanzer A, Djebali S, Tilgner H, Guernec G, Martin D, Merkel A, Knowles DG, Lagarde J, Veeravalli L, Ruan X, Ruan Y, Lassmann T, Carninci P, Brown JB, Lipovich L, Gonzalez JM, Thomas M, Davis CA, Shiekhattar R, Gingeras TR, Hubbard TJ, Notredame C, Harrow J, Guigo R (2012) The GENCODE v7 catalog of human long noncoding RNAs: analysis of their gene structure, evolution, and expression. Genome Res 22(9):1775–1789. https://doi.org/10.1101/gr.132159.111

7. Cabili MN, Trapnell C, Goff L, Koziol M, Tazon-Vega B, Regev A, Rinn JL (2011)

Integrative annotation of human large intergenic noncoding RNAs reveals global properties and specific subclasses. Genes Dev 25 (18):1915–1927. https://doi.org/10.1101/gad.17446611

8. Guttman M, Amit I, Garber M, French C, Lin MF, Feldser D, Huarte M, Zuk O, Carey BW, Cassady JP, Cabili MN, Jaenisch R, Mikkelsen TS, Jacks T, Hacohen N, Bernstein BE, Kellis M, Regev A, Rinn JL, Lander ES (2009) Chromatin signature reveals over a thousand highly conserved large non-coding RNAs in mammals. Nature 458 (7235):223–227. https://doi.org/10.1038/nature07672

9. Zhang Y, Wagner EK, Guo X, May I, Cai Q, Zheng W, He C, Long J (2016) Long intergenic non-coding RNA expression signature in human breast cancer. Sci Rep 6:37821. https://doi.org/10.1038/srep37821

10. Soreq L, Guffanti A, Salomonis N, Simchovitz A, Israel Z, Bergman H, Soreq H (2014) Long non-coding RNA and alternative splicing modulations in Parkinson's leukocytes identified by RNA sequencing. PLoS Comput Biol 10(3):e1003517. https://doi.org/10.1371/journal.pcbi.1003517

11. Ulitsky I, Bartel DP (2013) lincRNAs: genomics, evolution, and mechanisms. Cell 154 (1):26–46. https://doi.org/10.1016/j.cell.2013.06.020

12. Quinn JJ, Chang HY (2016) Unique features of long non-coding RNA biogenesis and function. Nat Rev Genet 17(1):47–62. https://doi.org/10.1038/nrg.2015.10

13. Iyer MK, Niknafs YS, Malik R, Singhal U, Sahu A, Hosono Y, Barrette TR, Prensner JR, Evans JR, Zhao S, Poliakov A, Cao X, Dhanasekaran SM, Wu YM, Robinson DR, Beer DG, Feng FY, Iyer HK, Chinnaiyan AM (2015) The landscape of long noncoding RNAs in the human transcriptome. Nat Genet 47 (3):199–208. https://doi.org/10.1038/ng.3192

14. Liu SJ, Nowakowski TJ, Pollen AA, Lui JH, Horlbeck MA, Attenello FJ, He D, Weissman JS, Kriegstein AR, Diaz AA, Lim DA (2016) Single-cell analysis of long non-coding RNAs in the developing human neocortex. Genome Biol 17:67. https://doi.org/10.1186/s13059-016-0932-1

15. Xie C, Yuan J, Li H, Li M, Zhao G, Bu D, Zhu W, Wu W, Chen R, Zhao Y (2014) NONCODEv4: exploring the world of long non-coding RNA genes. Nucleic Acids Res 42 (Database issue):D98–103. https://doi.org/10.1093/nar/gkt1222

16. Dobin A, Davis CA, Schlesinger F, Drenkow J, Zaleski C, Jha S, Batut P, Chaisson M, Gingeras TR (2013) STAR: ultrafast universal RNA-seq aligner. Bioinformatics 29(1):15–21. https://doi.org/10.1093/bioinformatics/bts635

17. Leinonen R, Sugawara H, Shumway M, International Nucleotide Sequence Database C (2011) The sequence read archive. Nucleic Acids Res 39(Database issue):D19–D21. https://doi.org/10.1093/nar/gkq1019

18. Andrews S (2010) FastQC: a quality control tool for high throughput sequence data. Available at: https://www.bioinformatics.babraham.ac.uk/projects/fastqc/

19. Krueger F (2015) A wrapper tool around Cutadapt and FastQC to consistently apply quality and adapter trimming to FastQ files. Available at: https://www.bioinformatics.babraham.ac.uk/projects/trim_galore/

20. Martin M (2011) Cutadapt removes adapter sequences from high-throughput sequencing reads. EMBnet J 17:10–12. https://doi.org/10.14806/ej.17.1.200

21. Li H, Handsaker B, Wysoker A, Fennell T, Ruan J, Homer N, Marth G, Abecasis G, Durbin R, Genome Project Data Processing S (2009) The sequence alignment/map format and SAMtools. Bioinformatics 25 (16):2078–2079. https://doi.org/10.1093/bioinformatics/btp352

22. Trapnell C, Williams BA, Pertea G, Mortazavi A, Kwan G, van Baren MJ, Salzberg SL, Wold BJ, Pachter L (2010) Transcript assembly and quantification by RNA-Seq reveals unannotated transcripts and isoform switching during cell differentiation. Nat Biotechnol 28(5):511–515. https://doi.org/10.1038/nbt.1621

23. Wang L, Park HJ, Dasari S, Wang S, Kocher JP, Li W (2013) CPAT: coding-potential assessment tool using an alignment-free logistic regression model. Nucleic Acids Res 41(6):e74. https://doi.org/10.1093/nar/gkt006

24. Finn RD, Coggill P, Eberhardt RY, Eddy SR, Mistry J, Mitchell AL, Potter SC, Punta M, Qureshi M, Sangrador-Vegas A, Salazar GA, Tate J, Bateman A (2016) The Pfam protein families database: towards a more sustainable future. Nucleic Acids Res 44(D1):D279–D285. https://doi.org/10.1093/nar/gkv1344

25. Trapnell C, Pachter L, Salzberg SL (2009) TopHat: discovering splice junctions with RNA-Seq. Bioinformatics 25(9):1105–1111. https://doi.org/10.1093/bioinformatics/btp120

26. Roberts A, Pimentel H, Trapnell C, Pachter L (2011) Identification of novel transcripts in annotated genomes using RNA-Seq. Bioinformatics 27(17):2325–2329. https://doi.org/10.1093/bioinformatics/btr355

27. Kong L, Zhang Y, Ye ZQ, Liu XQ, Zhao SQ, Wei L, Gao G (2007) CPC: assess the protein-coding potential of transcripts using sequence features and support vector machine. Nucleic Acids Res 35(Web Server issue):W345–W349. https://doi.org/10.1093/nar/gkm391

28. Love MI, Huber W, Anders S (2014) Moderated estimation of fold change and dispersion for RNA-seq data with DESeq2. Genome Biol 15(12):550. https://doi.org/10.1186/s13059-014-0550-8

29. Robinson MD, McCarthy DJ, Smyth GK (2010) edgeR: a Bioconductor package for differential expression analysis of digital gene expression data. Bioinformatics 26(1):139–140. https://doi.org/10.1093/bioinformatics/btp616

Chapter 11

Analysis of RNA-Seq Data Using TEtranscripts

Ying Jin and Molly Hammell

Abstract

Transposable elements (TE) are mobile genetic elements that can readily change their genomic position. When not properly silenced, TEs can contribute a substantial portion to the cell's transcriptome, but are typically ignored in most RNA-seq data analyses. One reason for leaving TE-derived reads out of RNA-seq analyses is the complexities involved in properly aligning short sequencing reads to these highly repetitive regions. Here we describe a method for including TE-derived reads in RNA-seq differential expression analysis using an open source software package called TEtranscripts. TEtranscripts is designed to assign both uniquely and ambiguously mapped reads to all possible gene and TE-derived transcripts in order to statistically infer the correct gene/TE abundances. Here, we provide a detailed tutorial of TEtranscripts using a published qPCR validated dataset.

Key words RNA-seq, Transposable elements, TEtranscripts, Differential expression analysis, STAR, DESeq

1 Introduction

1.1 Transposable Elements

Barbara McClintock laid the foundation for TE research with her discoveries in maize of mobile genetic elements capable of inserting into novel locations in the genome, altering the expression of nearby genes [1]. Since then, our appreciation of the contribution of repetitive TE-derived sequences to eukaryotic genomes has vastly increased. With the publication of the first human genome draft by the Human Genome Project, it was determined that nearly half of the human genome is derived from TE sequences [2, 3], with varying levels of repetitive DNA present in most plant and animal species. More recent studies looking at distantly related TE-like sequences have estimated that up to two thirds of the human genome might be repeat-derived [4], with the vast majority of these sequences attributed to retrotransposons that require transcription as part of the mobilization process, as discussed below.

Transposable elements are short DNA sequences (typically less than 10 kb) that can move from one genomic location to another. There are two main classes of TEs based on their "jumping"

Yejun Wang and Ming-an Sun (eds.), *Transcriptome Data Analysis: Methods and Protocols*, Methods in Molecular Biology, vol. 1751, https://doi.org/10.1007/978-1-4939-7710-9_11, © Springer Science+Business Media, LLC 2018

mechanism. Class-I elements, also named retroelements or retro-transposons, use a reverse transcriptase enzyme to copy an RNA transcript into the host DNA. Class-II elements, or DNA transposons, mainly move through a "cut and paste" mechanism involving the excision and reinsertion of the DNA sequence [5, 6]. Both classes are further subdivided to form a hierarchical classification system on the basis of the transposition mechanism, sequence similarities, and/or structural relationships [7]. It includes the levels of class, subclass, order, superfamily, family, subfamily, and insertion. Class, subclass, and order are defined according to the replication strategies. Superfamilies are distinguished by structures of protein or noncoding domains, such as the L1 and L2 subfamilies of LINE retrotransposons. Family/subfamily is defined on DNA sequence conservation. TEs in the same families share high levels of sequence similarity and are relatively distinct from other TE families. "Insertion" represents each genomic copy of a particular TE subfamily. For example, Repbase [8] and RepeatMasker [9] report 16,293 insertions for the L1Md_A subfamily in the mouse reference genome (mm9), all of which are more similar to each other than they are to other subfamilies of the L1 family (such as L1Md T).

Transposable elements propagate by multiplying within the genomes of host cells, and can be passed from generation to generation if a particular new insertion occurs in the germ line cell lineage. While the vast majority of TE copies are nonfunctional for mobilization; a very small subset has retained the ability to mobilize and occur as polymorphic insertions within the human population [10–16]. In addition, many nonmobile elements still contain functional regulatory information that can direct their transcription. While only retrotransposons require an RNA intermediate to transpose, both DNA and RNA transposons can be transcribed from the genome, and these TE-derived transcripts have been shown to accumulate in various conditions such as cancer [17–23] and neurodegenerative diseases [24–26]. Abundant TE transcripts have also been detected during certain stages of normal embryogenesis [27–29], neural development [30–35], and aging [24, 36, 37].

1.2 TEtranscripts

With the recent advances in next-generation sequencing technologies (NGS), it becomes possible to interrogate previously intractable questions, such as the genome-wide expression of these selfish genetic elements using RNA-seq assays. Many tools have been developed to analyze RNA-seq data. However, TE-associated reads are often discarded in sequencing data analyses because of the uncertainty in attributing ambiguously mapped reads to these regions, despite some previous attempts to integrate them in downstream analyses [38–43].

TEtranscripts [44] allows users to analyze both gene- and TE-associated reads concurrently in one simplified workflow. TEtranscripts estimates both gene and TE transcript abundances and conducts differential expression analysis on the resultant gene/TE abundance count table.

TEtranscripts is a reference-genome-based RNA-seq analysis tool. There are three main steps in standard RNA-seq analysis: mapping reads to a reference genome or transcriptome, estimating relative transcript abundance, and performing statistical differential expression analysis. TEtranscripts focuses on the last two steps (abundance estimation and differential expression). However, we provide extensive guidance on choosing appropriate alignment software that shows the least bias against detection of TE-derived reads.

2   Materials

TEtranscripts runs on the Linux command line. In the following description, commands are shown with a "$" prefix.

For the system requirements of running the software, please refer to analysis of running time and memory usage of TEtranscripts on simulated data shown in Table 1. A variety of library sizes ranging from 20 million to 80 million reads were generated based on the mouse genome (mm9), with each sample having 10% of the reads coming from TEs. While TEtranscripts takes additional time and memory to distribute reads between the millions of TE instances in the genome as compared to standard gene expression analysis packages, it is still relatively efficient, with a typical memory requirement of 8GB and run times on the order of 1–2.5 h for datasets with 20–100 million reads per sample. These calculations were all performed on a server with 128 GB memory and Xeon E5-2665 processors running at 2.40 GHz (16 cores). In general, we recommend using a 64-bit version of operating system.

2.1   Installation of the Software and Dependencies

TEtranscripts requires python 2.6.x or python 2.7.x, pysam 0.8.2.1, R 2.15 or greater, samtools 0.1.19 [45], and DESeq 1.5. x or greater. To map RNA-seq reads to a reference genome or transcriptome, we recommend to use STAR 2.5.2b or higher [46].

Table 1
Running time and memory usage

Sample size (million reads)	Time (h)	Memory (GB)
20	0.3030	7.819
40	0.7197	9.580
80	2.1320	11.463

We tested TEtranscripts on a set of simulated RNA-seq data with various mean sample sizes

In this demonstration, we have created several folders under the user's home directory ($HOME) to save source codes of tools, dependencies, and test data. All the software and libraries have been installed under $HOME, and we have added $HOME/bin and $HOME/lib/python2.7/site-packages to PATH and PYTHON-PATH environment variables respectively.

Download   pysam   from   https://github.com/pysam-developers/pysam/archive/0.8.1.tar.gz, put it into a folder labeled *Tools*. Unpack it and then install it into the user's home directory.

```
$mkdir ~/Tools
$cd Tools
$tar xvfz 0.8.1.tar.gz
$cd pysam-0.8.1
$ python setup.py install --prefix=$HOME
```

SAMtools (Sequence Alignment Map Tools) [45] version 0.1.19 can be downloaded from https://sourceforge.net/projects/samtools/files/samtools/0.1.19/. Download the tar ball to *Tools* and decompress it and install it to user's home directory.

```
$cd Tools
$tar xvfj samtools-0.1.19.tar.bz2
$cd samtools-0.1.19
$make
```

Copy *samtools* and/or other binaries into the *bin* folder under user's home directory.

```
$cp samtools $HOME/bin
```

TEtranscripts can be downloaded from http://hammelllab.labsites.cshl.edu/software.

Download the tar ball, decompress it and install it to user's home directory.

```
$cd Tools
$tar xvfz TEToolkit_1.5.1.tar.gz
$cd TEToolkit_1.5.1
$python setup.py install --prefix=$HOME
```

If all dependencies and tools have been installed correctly, the following command shows the help menu of TEtranscripts.

```
$TEtranscripts -h
```

STAR [46] source code and binaries can be downloaded from https://github.com/alexdobin/STAR/releases. The precompiled STAR executables are located in the *bin* subdirectory. From the unpacked STAR folder, copy the binaries to the bin folder under the user's home directory.

```
$cd Tools
$ tar xvfz 2.5.2b.tar.gz
$ cd STAR-2.5.2b
$cp bin/Linux_x86_64/STAR $HOME/bin
```

2.2 Example Dataset

For the purpose of this demonstration, we have chosen a published study involving the regulation of transposons in the *Drosophila melanogaster* genome. Ohtani and colleagues observed the derepression of transposable elements upon alteration of DmGTSF1, which works with the Piwi-associated silencing complex (piRISC) to silence TEs in the Drosophila ovary [47]. We have obtained the raw FASTQ reads from the National Center for Biotechnology Information (NCBI) Gene Expression Omnibus (accession no. GSE47006, https://www.ncbi.nlm.nih.gov). We have selected Piwi knockdown and control samples (GSM1142845 and GSM1142844). A folder called *Test_data* has been used to hold all test data and results.

```
$mkdir ~/Test_data
$mv piwi_KD.fastq.gz control_KD.fastq.gz ~/Test_data
```

Here, *piwi_KD.fastq.gz* and *control_KD.fastq.gz* represent the raw sequencing file names of Piwi knockdown and control samples.

2.3 Reference Genome and Annotation Files

The input data for TEtranscripts consists of alignment files in either the SAM or BAM format, and two annotation files in the General Transfer Format (GTF) ((http://mblab.wustl.edu/GTF22.html) for genes and TEs, respectively. For the purposes of this demonstration, we will use the terms "unique-reads" and "multi-reads" to designate the reads that have a unique alignment in the genome or map to multiple loci with equal quality, respectively. The utilization of multi-reads for TE quantification is critical, as a read originating from a TE could align to multiple instances (insertions) of that element in the genome. STAR supports multi-reads alignments, and provides limits for the maximum number of multiple alignments to report per read. In order to map RNA-seq reads, STAR needs an index file of the reference genome and transcriptome. We have downloaded the reference sequences and the gene annotation file of *Drosophila melanogaster* (dm3) from the UCSC genome database [48]. We have saved the index files in a folder named Index.

```
$mkdir ~/Index
$cp gene_ann.gtf ~/Index
$cp dm3.fa ~/Index
```

Here, *gene_ann.gtf* and *dm3.fa* represent the gene annotation file and the reference genome sequence file respectively. Both of them have been saved in a folder called *Index*.

The GTF file of transposable element annotation has been generated from the RepeatMasker table obtained from the UCSC genome database [48] and saved to the folder *Index*. The transposon annotation tables have been parsed to filter out low complexity and simple repeats, as well as non-TE structural and other small RNAs (rRNA, scRNA, snRNA, srpRNA, and tRNA). Each TE insertion in the table has been given a unique identifier. The genomic location, element name, as well as family and class information has been also extracted from the table and included in the GTF file (*see* **Note 1**). TEtranscripts can also utilize custom TE annotations, such as those generated from de novo TE insertion calls, as long as they conform to the format described above and are consistent with the genome sequencing files used for the alignment.

```
$cp TE_ann.gtf ~/Index
```

Once each of the annotation files is in place, one can use STAR to generate a genome index file to be used when aligning reads in the next step:

```
$ STAR --sjdbOverhang 100 --sjdbGTFfile ~/Index/gene_ann.gtf
--runMode genomeGenerate --genomeDir ~/Index --genomeFasta-
Files ~/dm3.fa --runThreadN 4
```

The option –runThreadN defines the number of threads running in parallel, and should be set according to the number of available cores on the server or desktop being used.

3   Methods

3.1   Running STAR to Map Raw RNA-Seq Reads

In order to recover reads originated from TEs, we have run our alignment software with the parameters set to report the best alignments for each read. For uniquely mappable reads, this will output 1 alignment per read. For ambiguously mapped reads, this will output all "equally likely" alignments, which in practice means all alignments with the same quality score for mappability. STAR has two parameters that play the most important role in the reporting of multi-mappers:

```
--winAnchorMultimapNmax
```

and

```
--outFilterMultimapNmax
```

(*see* **Note 2**).

Type the following commands to map the raw RNA-seq fastq files located in Test_data to the reference genome.

```
$cd ~/Test_data
$STAR --runThreadN 12 --genomeDir ~/Index/ --sjdbGTFfile ~/In-
dex/gene_ann.gtf  --sjdbOverhang 100  --readFilesIn  piwi_KD.
fastq.gz --readFilesCommand zcat --outSAMtype BAM Unsorted --
winAnchorMultimapNmax 200 --outFilterMultimapNmax 100 --out-
FileNamePrefix ~/Test_data/piwiKD_

$ STAR --runThreadN 12 --genomeDir ~/Index/ --sjdbGTFfile
~/Index/gene_ann.gtf --sjdbOverhang 100 --readFilesIn control_KD.
fastq.gz --readFilesCommand zcat --outSAMtype BAM Unsorted --winAn-
chorMultimapNmax 200 --outFilterMultimapNmax 100 --outFileName-
Prefix ~/Test_data/control_
```

If the input FASTQ files have been previously uncompressed, remove the "--readFilesCommand zcat" option. The previous commands allows STAR to output reads with at most 100 multiple alignments, defined by --outFilterMultimapNmax 100. To be able to find all of those alignments, STAR is set to use as many as 200 loci anchors. We have found that reporting a maximum of 100 alignments per read provides an optimal compromise between the size of the alignment file and the recovery of multi-mappers in this example dataset. However, we highly suggest that users optimize this parameter for their particular genomic TE content, as this could significantly improve the quality of transposable element quantification. To optimally set this parameter, we recommend a saturation analysis on the multi-read alignments (*see* **Note 3**).

The successful run will create a set of output files for both Piwi knockdown and control samples in the same folder Test_data, but with different prefix, piwiKD_ and control_ respectively. Files with a suffix of Aligned.out.bam are the main output files containing compressed alignment results from STAR.

3.2 Running TEtranscripts

Using the alignment files obtained from the previous step, now we can run TEtranscripts to estimate gene/TE abundances and conduct differential expression analysis.

```
$cd ~/Test_data
$ TEtranscripts --format BAM --stranded reverse -t piwiKD_
Aligned.out.bam -c control_Aligned.out.bam --GTF ~/Index/gen-
e_ann.gtf --TE ~/Index/TE_ann.gtf --mode multi --project pi-
wiKD_vs_control --minread 1 -i 10 --padj 0.05
```

TEtranscripts accepts alignment files in either SAM or BAM format. When there are multiple samples, for example biological replicates in one or both conditions, users can input all of them into one TEtranscripts run. Replicate samples of the same condition should be input together as a group and separated by a space. For example, a command with biological replicates included would look like:

```
$ TEtranscripts --format BAM --stranded reverse -t piwiKD_1_
Aligned.out.bam piwiKD_2_Aligned.out.bam -c control_1_
Aligned.out.bam control_2_Aligned.out.bam --GTF ~/Index/gene_
ann.gtf --TE ~/Index/TE_ann.gtf --mode multi --project
piwiKD_vs_control --minread 1 -i 10 --padj 0.05
```

TEtranscripts always performs pairwise comparisons, represented by the options -t (treatment) and -c (control). Additional comparisons should be performed as separate runs of TEtranscripts.

By default, TEtranscripts assumes that alignments are sorted by read names and not by coordinates, the default output for STAR. In other words, all alignments coming from one read should appear as consecutive rows in the file. However, if the alignment files were sorted by coordinates, the user can set the option –sortByPos (*see* **Note 4**), to direct TEtranscripts to resort the data files.

TEtranscripts provides two running modes: uniq and multi. Using uniq mode, only unique reads will be counted (including only uniquely mappable TE content), while multi-mode will take into account both unique reads and ambiguously mapped reads. We strongly recommend multi-mode for TE analysis.

TEtranscripts also supports strand-specific read counting, and applies it to both genes and TEs, with the option --stranded.

For single-end RNA-seq data, users can provide the average fragment length used for sequencing with the option -L. In the case of paired-end data, TEtranscripts will estimate this length from the input alignment file. This parameter is optional and not required.

Users can choose three different normalization approaches for differential analysis using the option —norm. Total annotated read counts (TC) will output RPM-like abundance estimates normalized to all mapped and annotated reads. Quantile normalization (quant) will normalize all samples to the quantiles of the average of all samples. Default DESeq [49] normalization (DESeq_default) will normalize each sample by the geometric mean of the annotated reads across all samples. Published comparisons of RNA-seq analysis protocols have favored DESeq-like normalization strategies, but we leave this option up to the user [50].

TEtranscripts uses an expectation-maximization (EM) algorithm to determine the maximum-likelihood estimates of multi-reads assignments to all TE transcripts. Briefly, we assume that truly transcribed TEs will contain reads across the entire length of the TE locus, while nontranscribed TEs will only contain reads at regions of high sequence similarity to other family members. Therefore, we redistribute reads upon each iteration of the EM loop towards highly expressed TEs with extensive read pileup along the locus. In practice, this EM loop usually converges within ten iterations (the default). Users can optionally specify the maximum number of iterations of the EM procedure, using the option -i.

Following gene and TE abundance estimation, TEtranscripts next calculates differential expression estimates for the two conditions being compared using the DESeq software package. The option --minread defines the minimum read count cutoff used to filter data for statistical analysis with DESeq. This is often useful in preventing nontranscribed TEs and genes from inflating the type I error correction calculations (also referred to as FDR, or false discovery rates). TEtranscripts returns two output tables from DESeq: the standard output table of fold change and p-value statistics for all genes and TEs, as well as a second table of only those genes and TEs calculated to be statistically significant in their differential expression between conditions. The option "--padj" is used to determine the minimum adjusted p-value considered as "significant," with a default value of $p < 0.05$.

3.3 Results

A successful TEtranscripts run will generate the following output files:

```
piwiKD_vs_control.cntTable, piwiKD_vs_control_DESeq.R,
piwiKD_vs_control_gene_TE_analysis.txt
piwiKD_vs_control_sigdiff_gene_TE.txt.
```

piwiKD_vs_control.cntTable contains the estimated raw abundance counts for all genes and TEs as a tab-delimited table. Each row represents a gene or TE, each column is a sample, and each value is a raw count.

piwiKD_vs_control_DESeq.R is an R script used by TEtranscripts for differential expression analysis. Users can use optionally use this script to rerun just the differential analysis portion of TEtranscripts with different settings. For example, the user may wish to alter the false discovery rate cutoff or to choose a different normalization approach. Rerunning just the differential expression portion of the analysis is much more efficient than rerunning the entire TEtranscripts software package.

piwiKD_vs_control_gene_TE_analysis.txt contains the differential expression results from DESeq for all genes and TEs.

piwiKD_vs_control_sigdiff_gene_TE.txt contains a subset of the differential expression analysis table for only those genes and TEs that passed the P-value significance criteria.

Here we present several plots of the analysis results using the included test data. For all of these figures, the data was taken from a

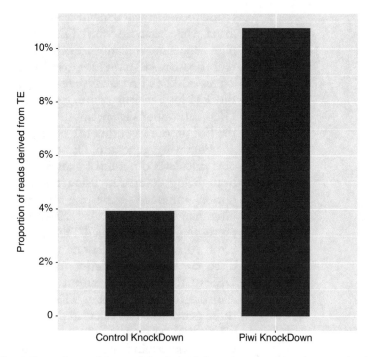

Fig. 1 Percentage of transcripts derived from transposable elements in the example datasets used in this protocol. The data presented was collected from Drosophila ovaries with either dsRNA targeting Piwi or a control nontargeting construct [47], while gene and TE expression analysis was performed with TEtranscripts

published study [47], but reanalyzed with the TEtranscripts software package.

Figure 1 shows the proportion of transcripts originating from transposable elements in the test datasets used for this protocol. Piwi knockdown samples (column 1) show a significant increase as compared to control samples with nontargeting dsRNA. Since Piwi is known to contribute to general TE regulation, many TEs are expected to show some increase in the Piwi knockdown samples, and this is reflected by an increase in the overall TE content of the expression library.

Figure 2 displays a scatter plot of the expression profiles of all genes and TEs for the Piwi knockdown and control samples for the same dataset described above. Here, we see that few protein-coding genes show substantial change in the Piwi knockdown samples (black dots), while most TEs show some degree of upregulation (red dots). This pattern is in line with the expected role of Piwi proteins as a general TE regulatory factor.

Figure 3 shows the estimated fold changes in TE levels as calculated by TEtranscripts as compared to q-PCR validation measurements of a selection of TEs from the dataset used in this protocol. The log2 fold change (log2FC) calculated by

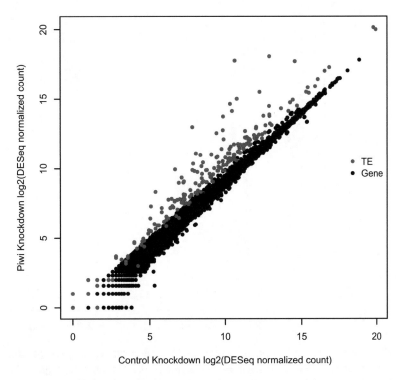

Fig. 2 Gene expression profiles of genes (black) and TEs (red) comparing Piwi knockdown and control samples. Nearly all TEs show upregulation in the Piwi knockdown samples as compared to controls. Data from [47] as previously described

TEtranscripts (green bars) closely resembles the measured q-PCR results (red bars) for most of the TEs interrogated. In addition, TEtranscripts correctly identifies TEs not expressed in these samples.

4 Notes

1. *Creating a TE GTF file.*
   We have created TE GTF files for several model organisms, such as human, mouse, maize, Drosophila, and Arabidopsis. They are freely available from http://hammelllab.labsites.cshl.edu/soft ware. Users can create their own TE GTF files for input to TEtranscripts, as long as the last field of the GTF file contains the following information about the TE instance: class, family, element, and unique instance id. As an example, for one insertion instance of the TE NINJA_I, we require the following annotation information:

```
gene_id "NINJA_I";
transcript_id "NINJA_I_dup1"; family_id "Pao";
class_id "LTR"
```

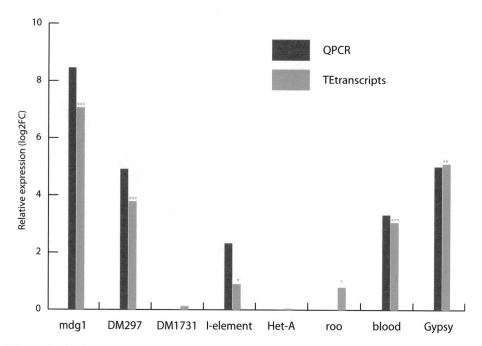

Fig. 3 Comparing TE fold change estimates from TEtranscripts to qPCR validation of the RNA-seq data. Log2 fold changes of Piwi knockdown versus control samples are shown in green for the TEtranscripts estimated fold change and in red for the qPCR measured fold change. The asterisk symbol represents the level of significance: "***" adjusted p-value $< 1e-5$, "**" adjusted p-value < 0.01, "*" adjusted p-value < 0.05. Data from [47] as previously described

All other information in the TE annotation file follows the standard GTF file format.

2. *Multi-reads output.*
   Many RNA-seq alignment packages support multi-reads alignments, and provide options to control for the maximum number of multiple alignments allowable per read. STAR has two parameters that play the most important role in the report of multi-mappers,

   ```
   --winAnchorMultimapNmax and
   ```

   ```
   --outFilterMultimapNmax.
   ```

   The author of STAR recommends setting.

   ```
   winAnchorMultimapNmax =2 * outFilterMultimapNmax
   ```

   (with a minimum value of 50). However, increasing winAnchorMultimapNmax allows STAR to use shorter seeds as anchors, which increases sensitivity for problematic alignments (with

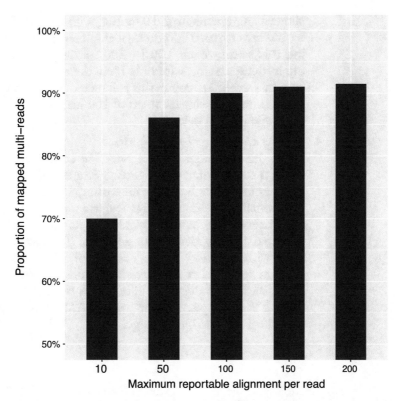

Fig. 4 Saturation analysis of multi-mapped reads. Once raising the limit on the number of reported alignments per read no longer substantially increases the overall mapping rates, we consider that most of the mappable reads have been recovered and the mappability rate has been "saturated." This rate varies depending upon the TE content of a given genome and the particular set of expressed TEs. The data presented here used a published mouse RNA-seq dataset examining the effects of TDP-43 loss [51]

many/mismatches indels). Therefore, users may need to test different combinations of these two parameters and to find the one that reports at least one alignment for most reads while maintaining high alignment qualities.

3. *Multi-reads saturation analysis.*

Here we show two examples for carrying out a saturation analysis to determine the optimal maximum number of allowable alignments per read. While we found that allowing 100 alignments was sufficient to detect most TE-derived reads in fly and mammalian genomes, other genomes may differ in: total genomic TE content, total number of insertions per TE, or relative sequence similarity between TE sub-families. Figure 4 shows an example of saturation analysis performed using a published mouse RNA-seq dataset (GSE27394) to identify transcriptional targets of the RNA-binding protein TDP-43 [51]. Using different cut-offs for the maximum alignments per read, from 10 to 200, we were able to show that the proportion of TE-derived reads detected increased dramatically when altering the maximal allowed alignments from 10 to 100, with 90% of all multi-reads having fewer than 100 potential alignments. However, increasing this setting from 100 to 200 maximal alignments shows diminishing returns, with only 1% of the remaining reads recovered by further increasing this parameter. Based on this analysis, we recommend using a cut-off of 100 maximum alignments for most mammalian datasets.

4. *Sorting alignments by coordinates.*
   When the alignment files are sorted by coordinates, users need to set the parameter –sortByPos. TEtranscripts will then resort the alignment files by read names using SAMtools. This is computationally time-consuming; we recommend using unsorted files, if available, since most alignment packages will output unsorted files by default. In addition, TEtranscripts may not work with the more recent versions of SAMtools, because of changes to the sort function. Therefore, we strongly recommend the use of alignment files sorted by read names prior to using TEtranscripts, and/or to use SAM tools version 0.1.19 with the TEtranscripts package.

References

1. McClintock B (1956) Controlling elements and the gene. Cold Spring Harb Symp Quant Biol 21:197–216

2. Lander ES, Linton LM, Birren B, Nusbaum C et al (2001) Initial sequencing and analysis of the human genome. Nature 409:860–921

3. Smit AF (1999) Interspersed repeats and other mementos of transposable elements in mammalian genomes. Curr Opin Genet Dev 9:657–663

4. de Koning AP, Gu W, Castoe TA, Batzer MA, Pollock DD (2011) Repetitive elements may comprise over two-thirds of the human genome. PLoS Genet 7(12):e1002384

5. Garfinkel DJ, Boeke JD, Fink GR (1985) Ty element transposition: reverse transcriptase and virus-like particles. Cell 42:507–517

6. Finnegan DJ (1989) Eukaryotic transposable elements and genome evolution. Trends Genet 5:103–107

7. Wicker T, Sabot F, Hua-Van A, Bennetzen JL et al (2007) A unified classification system for eukaryotic transposable elements. Nat Rev Genet 8:973–982

8. Jurka J et al (2005) Repbase update, a database of eukaryotic repetitive elements. Cytogent Genome Res 110:462–467

9. Smit A, et al. (1996–2010) Repeatmasker open-3.0. http://www.repeatmasker.org

10. Honma MA et al (1993) High-frequency germinal transposition of DsALS in Arabidopsis. Proc Natl Acad Sci U S A 90:6242–6246

11. Mills RE et al (2007) Which transposable elements are active in the human genome? Trends Genet 23:183–191

12. Bennett EA et al (2008) Active alu retrotransposons in the human genome. Genome Res 18:1875–1883

13. Kano H et al (2009) L1 retrotransposition occurs mainly in embryogenesis and creates somatic mosaicism. Genes Dev 23:1303–1312

14. Beck CR et al (2010) LINE-1 retrotransposition activity in human genomes. Cell 141:1159–1170

15. Hancks DC, Kazazian HH Jr (2012) Active human retrotransposons: variation and disease. Curr Opin Genet Dev 22:191–203

16. Huang CR et al (2012) Active transposition in genomes. Annu Rev Genet 46:651–675

17. Lamprecht B et al (2012) Derepression of an endogenous long terminal repeat activates the CSF1R proto-oncogene in human lymphoma. Nat Med 16:571–579

18. Lee E et al (2012) Landscape of somatic retrotransposition in human cancers. Science 337:967–971

19. Shukla R et al (2013) Endogenous retrotransposition activates oncogenic pathways in hepatocellular carcinoma. Cell 153:101–111

20. Sciamanna I et al (2013) A tumor-promoting mechanism mediated by retrotransposon-encoded reverse transcriptase is active in human transformed cell lines. Oncotarget 4:2271–2287

21. Criscione S et al (2014) Transcriptional landscape of repetitive elements in normal and cancer human cells. BMC Genomics 15:583

22. Sciamanna I et al (2014) Regulatory roles of LINE-1-encoded reverse transcriptase in cancer onset and progression. Oncotarget 5:8039–8051

23. Tubio JM et al (2014) Extensive transduction of nonrepetitive DNA mediated by L1 retrotransposition in cancer genomes. Science 345:1251343

24. Li W et al (2013) Activation of transposable elements during aging and neuronal decline in drosophila. Nat Neurosci 16:529–531

25. Reilly MT et al (2013) The role of transposable elements in health and diseases of the central nervous system. J Neurosci 33:17577–17586

26. Bundo M et al (2014) Increased L1 retrotransposition in the neuronal genome in schizophrenia. Neuron 81:306–313

27. Peaston AE et al (2004) Retrotransposons regulate host genes in mouse oocytes and preimplantation embryos. Dev Cell 7:597–606

28. Macia A et al (2011) Epigenetic control of retrotransposon expression in human embryonic stem cells. Mol Cell Biol 31:300–316

29. Fadloun A et al (2013) Chromatin signatures and retrotransposon profiling in mouse embryos reveal regulation of LINE-1 by RNA. Nat Struct Mol Biol 20:332–338

30. Muotri AR et al (2005) Somatic mosaicism in neuronal precursor cells mediated by L1 retrotransposition. Nature 35:903–910

31. Coufal NG et al (2009) L1 retrotransposition in human neural progenitor cells. Nature 460:1127–1131

32. Coufal NG et al (2011) Ataxia telangiectasia mutated (ATM) modulates long interspersed element-1 (l1) retrotransposition in human neural stem cells. Proc Natl Acad Sci U S A 108:20382–20387

33. Faulkner GJ et al (2009) The regulated retrotransposon transcriptome of mammalian cells. Nat Genet 41:563–571

34. Perrat PN et al (2013) Transposition-driven genomic heterogeneity in the Drosophila brain. Science 340:91–95

35. Thomas CA et al (2012) LINE-1 retrotransposition in the nervous system. Annu Rev Cell Dev Biol 28:555–573

36. De Cecco M et al (2013) Transposable elements become active and mobile in the genomes of aging mammalian somatic tissues. Aging 5:867–883

37. Sedivy JM et al (2013) Death by transposition – the enemy within? Bioessays 35:1035–1043

38. Rosenfeld JA et al (2009) Investigating repetitively matching short sequencing reads: the enigmatic nature of H3K9me3. Epigenetics 4:476–486

39. Day DS et al (2010) Estimating enrichment of repetitive elements from high-throughput sequence data. Genome Biol 11:R69

40. Wang J et al (2010) A Gibbs sampling strategy applied to the mapping of ambiguous short-sequence tags. Bioinformatics 26:2501–2508

41. Chung D et al (2011) Discovering transcription factor binding sites in highly repetitive regions of genomes with multiread analysis of ChIP-Seq data. PLoS Comput Biol 7: e1002111

42. Tucker BA et al (2011) Exome sequencing and analysis of induced pluripotent stem cells identify the cilia-related gene male germ cell-associated kinase (MAK) as a cause of retinitis pigmentosa. Proc Natl Acad Sci U S A 108: E569–E576

43. Treangen TJ, Salzberg SL (2011) Repetitive DNA and next-generation sequencing: computational challenges and solutions. Nat Rev Genet 13:36–46

44. Jin Y, Tam OH, Paniagua E, Hammell M (2015) TEtranscripts: a package for including transposable elements in differential expression analysis of RNA-seq datasets. Bioinformatics 31:3593–3599

45. Li H et al (2009) The sequence alignment/map format and SAMtools. Bioinformatics 25:2078–2079

46. Dobin A et al (2012) STAR: ultrafast universal RNA-seq aligner. Bioinformatics 29:15–21

47. Ohtani H et al (2013) DmGTSF1 is necessary for Piwi piRISC-mediated transcriptional transposon silencing in the drosophila ovary. Genes Dev 27:1656–1661

48. Karolchik D et al (2003) The UCSC genome browser database. Nucleic Acids Res 31:51–54

49. Anders S, Huber W (2010) Differential expression analysis for sequence count data. Genome Biol 11:R106

50. Lin Y, Golovnina K, Chen ZX, Lee HN et al (2016) Comparison of normalization and differential expression analysis using RNA-seq data from 726 individual Drosophila melanogaster. BMC Genomics 17:28

51. Polymenidou M et al (2011) Long pre-mRNA depletion and RNA missplicing contribute to neuronal vulnerability from loss of TDP-43. Nat Neurosci 14:459–468

Part III

New Applications of Transcriptome

Computational Analysis of RNA–Protein Interactions via Deep Sequencing

Lei Li, Konrad U. Förstner, and Yanjie Chao

Abstract

RNA-binding proteins (RBPs) function in all aspects of RNA processes including stability, structure, export, localization and translation, and control gene expression at the posttranscriptional level. To investigate the roles of RBPs and their direct RNA ligands in vivo, recent global approaches combining RNA immunoprecipitation and deep sequencing (RIP-seq) as well as UV-cross-linking (CLIP-seq) have become instrumental in dissecting RNA–protein interactions. However, the computational analysis of these high-throughput sequencing data is still challenging. Here, we provide a computational pipeline to analyze CLIP-seq and RIP-seq datasets. This generic analytic procedure may help accelerate the identification of direct RNA–protein interactions from high-throughput RBP profiling experiments in a variety of bacterial species.

Key words RNA-seq, RIP-seq, CLIP-seq, Bioinformatics, Hfq, CsrA, ProQ, ncRNA, sRNA

1 Introduction

RNA-binding proteins (RBPs) are an important class of post-transcriptional regulators of gene expression. RBPs either directly bind to messenger RNAs (mRNAs) or act through numerous regulatory noncoding RNAs (ncRNAs), dictating the fate of the bound transcripts. In all three kingdoms of life, increasing numbers of RBPs have been identified, including many well-studied model organisms such as pathogenic bacteria [1], baker's yeast [2], and human [3]. Taking bacteria for example, a new global RBP called ProQ was recently found as a major RNA chaperone in two distantly related bacterial pathogens *Salmonella enterica* serovar Typhimurium [1] and Legionella pneumophila [4], constituting the third global RBP in bacteria besides the well-known Hfq and CsrA proteins [5, 6].

Functional understanding of RBPs requires the full account of their RNA binding partners and the exact binding sites. To identify RNAs that are bound by an RBP of interest, a classic approach is to

Yejun Wang and Ming-an Sun (eds.), *Transcriptome Data Analysis: Methods and Protocols*, Methods in Molecular Biology, vol. 1751, https://doi.org/10.1007/978-1-4939-7710-9_12, © Springer Science+Business Media, LLC 2018

Table 1
Recent RNAseq-based studies of RNA–protein interactions in bacteria

Technique	Organism	RNA-binding protein	Year	PMID
RIP-seq	*Salmonella enterica* serovar Typhimurium	Hfq	2008	[7]
RIP-seq	*Salmonella enterica* serovar Typhimurium	Hfq	2012	[8]
RIP-seq	*Bacillus subtilis*	Hfq	2013	[10]
RIP-seq	*Sinorhizobium meliloti*	Hfq	2014	[11]
CLIP-seq	*Escherichia coli*	Hfq	2014	[12]
RIP-seq	*Escherichia coli*	Hfq	2014	[13]
RIP-seq	*Brucella suis*	Hfq	2015	[14]
RIP-seq	*Campylobacter jejuni*	CsrA	2016	[15]
CLIP-seq	*Salmonella enterica* serovar Typhimurium	Hfq, CsrA	2016	[16]
RIP-seq	*Salmonella enterica* serovar Typhimurium	ProQ	2016	[1]
RIP-seq	*Legionella pneumophila*	CsrA	2017	[17]
CLIP-seq	*Salmonella enterica* serovar Typhimurium	RNase E	2017	[18]

immunoprecipitate the RBP using a specific antibody followed by analysis of the copurified transcripts using RNA gels or DNA arrays (RIP-chip). Thanks to the advance of high-throughput sequencing technologies, unbiased deep sequencing of the co-immunoprecipitated RNAs (RIP-seq) can now identify hundreds or even thousands of transcripts in a bacterium [7, 8]. RIP-seq is relatively simple and experimentally straightforward, which have sparked its wide-application in the study of RNA–protein interactions in various biological systems [9] (Table 1). While RIP-seq usually identifies the full-length transcripts bound to an RBP, RIP-seq combined with UV cross-linking (CLIP-seq) can further identify the exact protein binding sites in a transcript. This approach was also referred to as HITS-CLIP, for high-throughput sequencing of RNA isolated by cross-linking immunoprecipitation [19]. The key of CLIP-seq is the in vivo cross-linking under ultraviolet (UV) light that introduces a covalent bond between RBP and the bound RNA. This covalent linkage enables the cross-linked RNA–protein complexes to survive stringent purification steps (often under denaturing conditions) and partial nuclease digestion to remove the unbound sequences. Deep sequencing of UV-cross-linked RNA fragments (CLIP-seq) informatively provides the locations of the protein-binding sites in a large number of transcripts [20]. The unique UV-cross-linking step makes CLIP-seq a powerful method to identify direct RNA–protein interactions. CLIP-seq has superior sensitivity in capturing weak or transient interactions in vivo [21]. In addition, the cross-linked peptide on RNA often results in mutations in cDNAs during reverse transcription. These mutations help pinpoint the exact protein-binding sites at the single nucleotide resolution [22].

This chapter mainly focuses on the CLIP-seq data analysis in bacteria, owing to its higher data complexity and its recent successful applications in *Escherichia coli* [12] and *S. Typhimurium* [16] (Table 1). In these studies, CLIP-seq has demonstrated its power in identifying the direct RNA ligands and exact sequences bound by Hfq and CsrA, respectively. While CLIP-seq is becoming instrumental in studying bacterial RNA–protein interactions, the analysis of CLIP-seq data is highly demanding. A suite of bioinformatics tools and analytic procedures are required to fully reveal the information capsulated in the sequencing data, and to identify the true RNA–protein interactions. To help other bioinformaticians and RNA enthusiasts perform such sequencing data analysis, here we have outlined a computational pipeline (Fig. 1) that has been recently devised to analyze CLIP-seq data for Hfq and CsrA [23]. Because these analytical procedures are generic, the presented pipeline can be readily used for the analysis of CLIP-seq with any given RBP, as well as the analysis of RIP-seq data.

2   Materials

We use our recently published CLIP-seq dataset [24] as an example, which is hosted in NCBI GEO database (GSE74425). The *S.* Typhimurium SL1344 reference genome and annotation information can be downloaded from NCBI FTP site (ftp://ftp.ncbi.nlm. nih.gov/genomes/archive/old_refseq/Bacteria/Salmonella_ enterica_serovar_Typhimurium_SL1344_uid86645/).

3   Methods

3.1   *Quality Trimming*

Upon completing the Illumina sequencing, the received raw sequencing reads require initial processing. A sequencing read must contain parts of the adapter sequences, which need be identified and trimmed before aligning to the reference genomes. Among many suitable tools, **Cutadapt** is a user-friendly command line interface. It can search and trim adapter sequences in an error-tolerant manner, and it is compatible with a large variety of input file formats generated by high-throughput sequencers [23] (*see* **Note 1**). The latest version can be downloaded from http:// cutadapt.readthedocs.io/en/stable/index.html.

To perform adaptor trimming for paired-end reads, a typical command line employing **Cutadapt** looks like this:

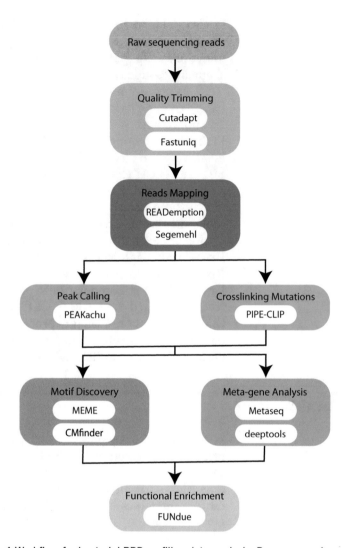

Fig. 1 Workflow for bacterial RBP profiling data analysis. Raw sequencing reads from CLIP-seq or RIP-seq are subjected to the analysis pipeline. Quality and user-defined sequence trimming removes adapter sequences, low-quality reads, and PCR duplicates using **Cutadapt** and **Fastuniq** tools. Reads are then mapped to the reference genome using **READemption** and **segemehl**. RBP-binding sites in RNA are identified using peak-calling algorithm **PEAKachu**, as well as the mutation analysis package **PIPE-seq**. The putative motifs sequences and structural properties are identified using **MEME** and **CMfinder**. Further, meta-gene analysis is performed using **Metaseq** and **deeptools** to search the global distribution of binding profiles. **FUNdue** finally reports a functional annotation including gene ontology and pathway analysis

```
cutadapt -q 20 -a "AGATCGGAAGAGCACACGTCTGAACTCCAGTCAC" -A
"GATCGTCGGACTGTAGAACTCTGAACGTGTAGATCTCGGTGGTCGCCGTATCATT"
--pair-filter=both -o [file1].out.fq -p [file2].out.fq
[file1].fq [file2].fq
```

The low-quality sequences from the end of short reads were firstly trimmed with a cutoff of 20 for the Phred quality score ($Q < 20$), then the two adapter sequences shown above were removed. This option (--pair-filter=both) removes the entire (pair-end sequenced) read pairs if at least one of the two sequences became shorter than a certain length threshold.

CLIP-seq experiments often generate numerous PCR duplicates after cDNA amplification. These duplicate reads need to be identified and removed using **Fastuniq** [24], a tool for de novo removal of duplicates in paired short reads and freely available at https://sourceforge.net/projects/fastuniq/.

3.2 Reads Mapping

The filtered and trimmed reads are then aligned against the reference genome using **READemption** [25]. **READemption** is a pipeline for the computational analysis of RNA-Seq data. It was developed initially for bacterial transcriptomic data, but now also extended to analyze eukaryotic transcriptomes as well as a mixture of both, i.e., dual RNA-Seq data [26]. The latest version can be downloaded from https://pythonhosted.org/READemption/. It requires **segemehl** [27] as the short read aligner, which can be download separately from http://www.bioinf.uni-leipzig.de/Software/segemehl/. **Segemehl** effectively handles both mismatches and short insertions and deletions. It is an ideal aligner for CLIP-seq reads, which often contain the characteristic mutations introduced by cross-linking procedures.

READemption covers most of the important mapping procedures and is organized in a command-line interface with several subcommands. These subcommands include read processing and aligning, coverage calculation, gene expression quantification, differential gene expression analysis as well as generating coverage files for visualization.

The *"create"* subcommand in **READemption** can generate the necessary folder structure. As required, transcriptome reads in FASTA format need be stored in the folder *input/reads*, and the genomes used as the reference should be in the folder *input/reference_sequences*. Also, the bacterial annotation files have to be placed into input/annotations.

After the initial folder setup, the subcommand for running the read alignment is

```
reademption align --realign, --processes 20 --segemehl_accuracy
95 --min_read_length 12 --progress [project_path]
```

Where [project_path] should be substituted by the path that was used with the *create* subsommand. Of note, reads shorter than 12 nucleotides will be removed, as well as the reads that are mapped to multiple locations. The remaining reads will then be aligned against the reference genome with a mapping accuracy of 95% using **segemehl**. The reads mapping statistics, including the summary of uniquely aligned reads and mapped reads, will be documented in the file read_alignment_stats.csv. The read alignment and index files will be generated in BAM and BAI format, respectively.

Reads coverage information representing the numbers of mapped reads per nucleotide can be generated using the "coverage" subcommand. The command line is

```
reademption coverage --unique_only [project_path]
```

The uniquely aligned reads will be used to generate the coverage file and saved in wiggle format. **READemption** also provides other useful options such as --coverage_style first_base_only, which converts only the first base into coverage files. This option is particularly useful to identify the transcript ends, which has served the analysis of global RNase E processing sites in our recent TIER-seq data [18]. The coverage plot can be visualized in a genome browser, e.g., the Integrated Genome Browser [28].

3.3 Peak Calling

RBP-binding sites in a transcript often accumulate many sequencing reads, which form sharp peaks spanning a narrow region. Therefore, peak calling serves to identify the precise RBP-binding sites, one of the most critical steps in the CLIP-seq data analysis. A few issues may influence the binding site detection. Firstly, most of the standard CLIP-seq protocols do not include a negative background control, which makes it hard to estimate the background noise and eliminate false peaks. This is because reads falling into a given transcript can be explained by two factors: transcript abundance and RBP preference, thus a negative control is highly recommended. Secondly, reads may align to incorrect transcripts due to sequencing errors and their subsequent mapping. A robust peak-calling algorithm is crucial to distinguish the specific RBP binding from nonspecific bindings and/or background noise. Although a few computational approaches have been developed, few are optimal because of problematic null hypotheses, e.g., **Piranha** [29], which considers sites with small number of reads as noise without including a negative control. A new peak-calling algorithm [16] has been developed to address these issues. This approach first divides the consecutively mapped reads into a few genomics blocks, and the blocks, which fulfill overlapping requirements including the read coverage of each block and the distance of the blocks, are iteratively assembled into the candidate peak regions using **blockbuster** [30]. Importantly, each candidate peak is tested for significant enrichment in the cross-linked samples versus the non-cross-linked control samples using **DESeq2** [31]. This algorithm will be integrated in a peak-calling tool **PEAKachu**, which is still under development, https://github.com/tbischler/PEAKachu (T. Bischler, personal communication).

3.4 Cross-Linking-Induced Mutations

Another important step is the identification of cross-linking induced mutations, which can be used to pinpoint the direct RNA–protein interaction sites at the single-nucleotide level. However, most of the available computational tools either ignore or inadequately address this issue, because the mutations may be confounded by single nucleotide polymorphisms (SNPs) and sequencing errors. One exception is **PIPE-CLIP** [32]. This tool can statistically identify the outstanding cross-linked mutations across a background distribution. Briefly, each mutation site is described by two parameters (k_i, m_i), where k_i is the number of mapped reads covering the considered location, and m_i is the number of specific mutations at location i. Then the mutation rate is modeled in each position by the binomial distribution with size k_i and background rate, which is calculated by read coverage with a summarization of matched length of all reads divided by genome size (*see* **Note 2**). The mutations will be considered significant only if the calculated adjusted p-value is lower than a specified threshold (e.g., adjusted $p < 0.05$). The source code of **PIPE-CLIP** is freely available from https://github.com/QBRC/PIPE-CLIP.

The command line for identifying cross-linking mutations is:

```
python pipeclip.py -i [inputfile] -o [output_prefix] -c 0 -l
12 -M 0.05 -C 0.05 -s [species]
```

The -c option is to specify the CLIP-seq type, -l option is to specify minimum match length, -M option is false discovery rate for significant cross-linking mutation, -C option defines the false discovery rate for the peak clusters.

For the paired-end reads, **PIPE-CLIP** cannot be directly used for mutation calling. However, there are a few solutions. First, the Python script 'FindMutation.py' can be used to identify substitutions, deletions and insertions separately from the mapping BAM files while allowing the user to choose the specific CLIP-seq type (HITS-CLIP, PAR-CLIP). Second, to lower the bias caused by background noise, the first read of the paired-reads can be extracted using **samtools** [33] and the characteristic mutation sites need to be present in both paired reads. Thirdly, the script 'MutationFilter.py' can determine the significantly enriched mutations in each library by using the extracted first paired mapping reads in BAM format and consensus mutation sites in BED format as input.

3.5 Motif Discovery

To investigate whether any sequence preference is present near the protein binding regions, **MEME** [34], a de novo sequence motif detection tool, can be used to discover consensus sequences among peak sequences or the surrounding regions of enriched cross-linking mutations. **MEME** can be accessed via a Web interface (http://meme-suite.org/tools/meme).

In addition to sequence-specific binding, some RBPs recognize RNA partners by structural properties rather than the sequence per se. **CMfinder** [35] is a tool that performed well to search for the presence of structural motifs based on unaligned sequences with long extraneous flanking regions. It relies on an expectation maximization algorithm using covariance models for motif description, and a Bayesian framework for structure prediction combining folding energy and sequence covariation. **CMfinder** can be accessed using webserver (http://wingless.cs.washington.edu/htbin-post/unrestricted/CMfinderWeb/CMfinderInput.pl). It is also available as a stand-alone perl script, which can be downloaded from http://bio.cs.washington.edu/CMfinderWeb/CMfinderInput.pl.

The command to run **CMfinder** is

```
perl cmfinder.pl [infile]
```

The output motif files are named by using the input file name as prefix (e.g., with the input file name input_file, the file input_file.motif.* will be generated). These motif files are stored in Stockholm format, where the suffix indicates the number of stem-loops in a motif. The motif file needs be reformatted to the unblocked Stockholm format. This is done with the **HMMER** package (http://hmmer.org/).

```
sreformat --pfam stockholm [alignfile] > [infile]
```

The formatted Stockholm file can be visualized using **R2R** [36], a software that generates representations of structure-informed RNA secondary alignments. The latest version is available at http://breaker.research.yale.edu/R2R.

3.6 Meta Gene Analysis

Meta gene analysis aims to analyze the global peak distribution with respect to a specific location across all annotated genes. The peak density can be calculated by counting the number of peaks along the specified annotation features like start codons, stop codons, sRNAs, and Rho-independent terminators. For example, a meta gene analysis of Hfq peaks found that most peaks are located at 3′ of seed sequences in sRNAs, whereas in mRNAs they are found at the 5′ of sRNA base-pairing regions [37].

A few computational tools are available for meta gene analysis. **Metaseq** [38] enables integrating multiple genomic data formats and allows for customized visualization. It is freely available at https://github.com/daler/metaseq. Another tool is **deepTools2** [39], which can jointly analyze multiple signals (bigWig) and region files (BED), and visualize data in a composite image. It is freely available at https://github.com/fidelram/deepTools and can also be used with a galaxy-based platform (http://deeptools.ie-freiburg.mpg.de/).

3.7 Functional Annotation and Enrichment Analysis

After the identification of RBP-binding sites, it is of interest to understand whether there is any enrichment of functions or pathways among the RBP-bound genes. To carry out this analysis in bacteria, we have developed a computational tool named **FUNdue** (L.L., unpublished). This tool is still under development (*see* **Note 3**) and is available at https://github.com/LeiLiSysBio/FUNdue.

FUNdue covers multiple submodules for functional ontologies and pathways analysis including gene ontology and pathway retrieval, functional assignment, statistics enrichment and visualization. Briefly, the gene ontology and pathway information is automatically retrieved from UniProt and KEGG databases. The ontology of each gene is classified into three categories, the molecular function, biological process and cellular component. Enrichment analysis is performed to evaluate the significant terms compared to the background using Fisher exact test and gene set enrichment analysis [40]. The calculated *p*-values are subjected to multiple-testing analysis using the Benjamini–Hochberg method. The significant gene ontology terms will be visualized as bar plots. Furthermore, the output files can be visualized by other tools such as **REVIGO** [37], which offers an easy and interactive illustration via web interface.

The following part demonstrates the steps for a pathway enrichment analysis using **FUNdue**. To initial a project and generate the required folder structure, we use the *"create"* submodule. The call to create the folder is:

```
traplfun create [project_path]
```

Where the [project_path] is the analysis folder specified by the user. This will result in a folder structure with all the required subfolders. **FUNdue** can automatically access and retrieve the pathways stored in the KEGG database [41], if the organism code is given. The three-letter organism code for a species of choice can be found on the KEGG website http://www.genome.jp/kegg/cata log/org_list.html. For example, if you want to download all the KEGG pathway information for *S.* Typhimurium SL1344 (organism code sey), the command is:

```
traplfun retrieve_pa -c sey [project_path]
```

After a list of interesting genes is created and stored in the *input/target_ids*, we can use the subcommand *'pathway_stat'* to perform enrichment analysis with default fisher exact test. The command is:

```
traplfun pathway_stat [project_path]
```

The significantly overrepresented pathways, per default with a *p*-value lower than 0.05, are stored in the pathway folder *output/pathway/pathwy_enrichment* in plain text format.

These pathways can then be visualized using the subcommand *'path_viz'*. The command is:

```
traplfun path_viz -c [KEGG_organism_code] [project_path]
```

It creates histograms and a bar plot for the enriched pathway summary. Besides the fisher exact test, the user can choose another gene set enrichment analysis [42], which maps and renders the changes in the relevant pathway graphs.

4   Notes

1. **READemption** can perform basic quality trimming and adapter clipping; however **cutadapt** has many advanced functions such as processing of paired-end sequencing reads, which is more suitable for CLIP-seq because the size of RBP interaction regions are comparable to whole cDNA fragments, and thus more accurately defines the binding regions.

2. Installation of **FUNdue** requires a few python and R dependent packages. This included Scipy, and also a few R packages including KEGGREST, getopt, piano, optparse, gsge, and pathview.

3. **PIPE-CLIP** can identify all simple types of mutations including substitutions, deletions and insertions. To avoid sequencing or alignment errors, each different type of mutation needs to be analyzed separately. UV-cross-linking mutations such as T to C mutations should be enriched at specific sites and show high frequency compared to other mutations. In addition, integrating the enriched mutations with peaks information could further pinpoint the cross-linking induced mutations.

Acknowledgment

We thank Erik Holmqvist and Andrew Camilli for critical reading and comments on the manuscript.

References

1. Smirnov A, Förstner KU, Holmqvist E et al (2016) Grad-seq guides the discovery of ProQ as a major small RNA-binding protein. Proc Natl Acad Sci U S A 113:11591–11596

2. Tsvetanova NG, Klass DM, Salzman J, Brown PO (2010) Proteome-wide search reveals unexpected RNA-binding proteins in Saccharomyces cerevisiae. PLoS One 5:pii:e12671

3. Castello A, Fischer B, Eichelbaum K et al (2012) Insights into RNA biology from an atlas of mammalian mRNA-binding proteins. Cell 149:1393–1406

4. Attaiech L, Boughammoura A, Brochier-Armanet C et al (2016) Silencing of natural transformation by an RNA chaperone and a multitarget small RNA. Proc Natl Acad Sci U

S A 113:8813–8818. https://doi.org/10.1073/pnas.1601626113

5. Vogel J, Luisi BF (2011) Hfq and its constellation of RNA. Nat Rev Microbiol 9:578–589. https://doi.org/10.1038/nrmicro2615

6. Romeo T (1998) Global regulation by the small RNA-binding protein CsrA and the non-coding RNA molecule CsrB. Mol Microbiol 29:1321–1330

7. Sittka A, Lucchini S, Papenfort K et al (2008) Deep sequencing analysis of small noncoding RNA and mRNA targets of the global post-transcriptional regulator, Hfq. PLoS Genet 4: e1000163

8. Chao Y, Papenfort K, Reinhardt R et al (2012) An atlas of Hfq-bound transcripts reveals 3′ UTRs as a genomic reservoir of regulatory small RNAs. EMBO J 31:4005–4019. https://doi.org/10.1038/emboj.2012.229

9. Riley KJ, Steitz JA (2013) The "observer effect" in genome-wide surveys of protein-RNA interactions. Mol Cell 49:601–604. https://doi.org/10.1016/j.molcel.2013.01.030

10. Dambach M, Irnov I, Winkler WC (2013) Association of RNAs with *Bacillus subtilis* Hfq. PLoS One 8:e55156. https://doi.org/10.1371/journal.pone.0055156

11. Torres-Quesada O, Reinkensmeier J, Schlüter JP et al (2014) Genome-wide profiling of Hfq-binding RNAs uncovers extensive post-transcriptional rewiring of major stress response and symbiotic regulons in *Sinorhizobium meliloti*. RNA Biol 11(5):563–579. https://doi.org/10.4161/rna.28239

12. Tree JJ, Granneman S, McAteer SP et al (2014) Identification of bacteriophage-encoded anti-sRNAs in pathogenic *Escherichia coli*. Mol Cell 55:199–213

13. Bilusic I, Popitsch N, Rescheneder P et al (2014) Revisiting the coding potential of the *E. coli* genome through Hfq co-immunoprecipitation. RNA Biol 11(5):641–654. https://doi.org/10.4161/rna.29299

14. Saadeh B, Caswell CC, Chao Y et al (2016) Transcriptome-wide identification of Hfq-associated RNAs in *Brucella suis* by deep sequencing. J Bacteriol 198:427–435. https://doi.org/10.1128/JB.00711-15

15. Dugar G, Svensson SL, Bischler T et al (2016) The CsrA-FliW network controls polar localization of the dual-function flagellin mRNA in *Campylobacter jejuni*. Nat Commun 7:11667

16. Holmqvist E, Wright PR, Li L et al (2016) Global RNA recognition patterns of post-transcriptional regulators Hfq and CsrA revealed by UV crosslinking in vivo. EMBO J

35:991–1011. https://doi.org/10.15252/embj.201593360

17. Sahr T, Rusniok C, Impens F et al (2017) The *Legionella pneumophila* genome evolved to accommodate multiple regulatory mechanisms controlled by the CsrA-system. PLoS Genet 13:e1006629. https://doi.org/10.1371/journal.pgen.1006629

18. Chao Y, Li L, Girodat D et al (2017) In vivo cleavage map illuminates the central role of RNase E in coding and non-coding RNA pathways. Mol Cell 65:39–51

19. Licatalosi DD, Mele A, Fak JJ et al (2008) HITS-CLIP yields genome-wide insights into brain alternative RNA processing. Nature 456:464–469. https://doi.org/10.1038/nature07488

20. König J, Zarnack K, Luscombe NM, Ule J (2011) Protein-RNA interactions: new genomic technologies and perspectives. Nat Rev Genet 13:77–83. https://doi.org/10.1038/nrg3141

21. Darnell RB (2010) HITS-CLIP: panoramic views of protein-RNA regulation in living cells. Wiley Interdisc Rev RNA 1:266–286. https://doi.org/10.1002/wrna.31

22. Zhang C, Darnell RB (2011) Mapping in vivo protein-RNA interactions at single-nucleotide resolution from HITS-CLIP data. Nat Biotechnol 29:607–614. https://doi.org/10.1038/nbt.1873

23. Martin M (2011) Cutadapt removes adapter sequences from high-throughput sequencing reads. EMBnet J 17:10. https://doi.org/10.14806/ej.17.1.200

24. Xu H, Luo X, Qian J et al (2012) FastUniq: a fast de novo duplicates removal tool for paired short reads. PLoS One 7:e52249

25. Förstner KU, Vogel J, Sharma CM (2014) READemption-a tool for the computational analysis of deep-sequencing-based transcriptome data. Bioinformatics 30:3421–3423

26. Westermann AJ, Förstner KU, Amman F et al (2016) Dual RNA-seq unveils noncoding RNA functions in host-pathogen interactions. Nature 529:496–501. https://doi.org/10.1038/nature16547

27. Hoffmann S, Otto C, Kurtz S et al (2009) Fast mapping of short sequences with mismatches, insertions and deletions using index structures. PLoS Comput Biol 5:e1000502

28. Freese NH, Norris DC, Loraine AE (2016) Integrated genome browser: visual analytics platform for genomics. Bioinformatics 32:2089–2095

29. Uren PJ, Bahrami-Samani E, Burns SC et al (2012) Site identification in high-throughput

RNA-protein interaction data. Bioinformatics 28:3013–3020. https://doi.org/10.1093/bio informatics/bts569

30. Langenberger D, Bermudez-Santana C, Hertel J et al (2009) Evidence for human microRNA-offset RNAs in small RNA sequencing data. Bioinformatics 25:2298–2301

31. Love MI, Huber W, Anders S (2014) Moderated estimation of fold change and dispersion for RNA-seq data with DESeq2. Genome Biol 15:550. https://doi.org/10.1186/PRE ACCEPT-8897612761307401

32. Chen B, Yun J, Kim MS et al (2014) PIPE-CLIP: a comprehensive online tool for CLIP-seq data analysis. Genome Biol 15:R18

33. Li H, Handsaker B, Wysoker A et al (2009) The sequence alignment/map format and SAMtools. Bioinformatics 25:2078–2079. https://doi.org/10.1093/bioinformatics/btp352

34. Bailey TL, Boden M, Buske FA et al (2009) MEME SUITE: tools for motif discovery and searching. Nucleic Acids Res 37:W202–W208

35. Yao Z, Weinberg Z, Ruzzo WL (2006) CMfinder—a covariance model based RNA motif finding algorithm. Bioinformatics 22:445–452

36. Weinberg Z, Breaker RR (2011) R2R—software to speed the depiction of aesthetic consensus RNA secondary structures. BMC Bioinformatics 12:3

37. Supek F, Bošnjak M, Škunca N, Šmuc T (2011) REVIGO summarizes and visualizes long lists of gene ontology terms. PLoS One 6:e21800

38. Dale RK, Matzat LH, Lei EP (2014) metaseq: a Python package for integrative genome-wide analysis reveals relationships between chromatin insulators and associated nuclear mRNA. Nucleic Acids Res 42:9158–9170

39. Ramírez F, Ryan DP, Grüning B et al (2016) deepTools2: a next generation web server for deep-sequencing data analysis. Nucleic Acids Res 44:W160–W165

40. Subramanian A, Tamayo P, Mootha VK et al (2005) Gene set enrichment analysis: a knowledge-based approach for interpreting genome-wide expression profiles. Proc Natl Acad Sci 102:15545–15550

41. Kanehisa M, Sato Y, Kawashima M et al (2016) KEGG as a reference resource for gene and protein annotation. Nucleic Acids Res 44: D457–D462

42. Luo W, Brouwer C (2013) Pathview: an R/bioconductor package for pathway-based data integration and visualization. Bioinformatics 29:1830–1831

Chapter 13

Predicting Gene Expression Noise from Gene Expression Variations

Xiaojian Shao and Ming-an Sun

Abstract

The level of gene expression is known to vary from cell to cell and even in the same cell over time. This variability provides cells with the ability to mitigate environmental stresses and genetic perturbations, and facilitates gene expression evolution. Recently, many valuable gene expression noise data measured at the single-cell level and gene expression variation measured for cell populations have become available. In this chapter, we show how to perform integrative analysis using these data. Specifically, we introduce how to apply a machine learning technique (support vector regression) to explore the relationship between gene expression variations and stochastic noise.

Key words Gene expression variation, Intrinsic noise, Single-cell, Machine learning, Feature selection, Support vector regression

1 Introduction

The phenomenon of stochastic fluctuation in protein abundance for a gene among single cells (gene expression noise) had been observed back to 1957 and it is thought to be inevitable. It is demonstrated that expression noise can contribute to drastically diverse phenotypes, even within isogenic (i.e., genetically identical) cell populations and under identical experimental conditions [1–3]. The gene expression noise could help cells to adapt to the environmental perturbation or external stresses [4–9]. Moreover, it is also evidenced that expression noise facilitates the evolution of gene regulation [4, 10–13]. Practically, expression noise can be divided into *intrinsic* and *extrinsic* categories. The *intrinsic* noise refers to the variation of expression level in identically regulated genes within a single cell, which could be generated from the inherent stochasticity of biochemical processes such as transcription and translation [1]. The *extrinsic* noise refers to variation of expression level in identically regulated genes from different cells or in a single cell over time [4, 14]. These expression noises can be

Yejun Wang and Ming-an Sun (eds.), *Transcriptome Data Analysis: Methods and Protocols*, Methods in Molecular Biology, vol. 1751, https://doi.org/10.1007/978-1-4939-7710-9_13, © Springer Science+Business Media, LLC 2018

quantified by attaching a fluorescently tagged reporter to a gene of interest, and measuring the distribution of fluorescence intensities over a population of clonal cells [14–18]. This allows us to distinguish *intrinsic* noise from *extrinsic* noise by using cell gating or orthogonal reporters.

Over the last few years, the origin and behaviour of such stochastic fluctuations of gene expression have been extensively characterized [1], yet still remain incompletely understood. Efforts using biochemistry experimental approaches, thermodynamic model and information theory have been made to better understand the molecular mechanism underlying noise in gene expression [19]. For example, gene regulatory networks are reported to contribute to expression noise which had also been simulated with thermodynamic models where a set of differential equations are used to describe the stochastic regulatory dynamics among genes [4, 20–24]. Other statistical models such as the Ω-expansion techniques are also used to investigate the translation bursting hypothesis, and pattern of stochastic fluctuations in a single-gene network with negative feedback regulation [25, 26]. For more details about these models, please refer to recent review [25].

However, all these theoretical models usually simulate the stochastic behavior of a single gene or a single-gene network but fail to model large systems consisting of multiple genes [4]. Recently, with the rapid development of single-cell and single-molecule based high-throughput techniques, large amount of gene expression variation data from single-cell (organism) have become available [27–33]. It provides us the opportunity to systematically investigate the relationship between expression noise and expression variation, which can improve our understanding of the variability and evolvability of gene expression. In this protocol, we will first delineate the relationship between gene expression noise and variation using correlation analysis, and then apply a machine-learning technique, the support vector regression (SVR) [34–37], to fit the relationship between them. We will show gene expression variations are predictive for noise level, which imply common mechanisms underlying both gene expression noise and variations. Particularly, we will focus on data from a single-cell organism—budding yeast (*S. cerevisiae*) as an example to demonstrate this protocol.

2   Materials

2.1   Gene Expression Noise Data

Large-scale *expression noise* data of single cells were obtained from the study by Newman et al. [17]. This data measures the protein abundances of 4159 genes on a collection of budding yeast (*S. cerevisiae*) strains in rich media (YEPD) using high-throughput flow cytometry. The coefficient of variation (CV, i.e., standard deviation/mean) was used to measure the differences of protein abundances from cell to cell. In order to control the confounding influences from protein abundance, or from the instrument response or the intracellular differences in cells, the distance of each CV to a median of CV values (i.e., named as DM value) were calculated. Both CV profiles and DM profiles could be extracted from the Supplementary Table 1 of [17].

2.2 Gene Expression Variation Data

Gene expression variation is defined as the variance of given genes' expressions across different conditions. These gene expressions could be measured using any transcriptome profiling approaches such as microarray or RNA-Seq. Here the gene expression variation data mainly contain five different types: (1) expression variation under different environmental conditions; (2) expression variation under genetic perturbations of *trans*-acting factors; (3) expression variations among individuals, and among isolates yielded by mutational accumulation; (4) expression divergence of orthologous genes between related strains; or (5) related species. All these data could be downloaded from respective studies.

We further compiled 633 microarray datasets from Gene Expression Omnibus (GEO, http://www.ncbi.nlm.nih.gov/geo/) with accessions: GSE18, GSE20, GSE21, GSE22, GSE23, GSE24, GSE25, GSE26, GSE28, GSE29, GSE2239, GSE2953, GSE2977, GSE3182, GSE3358, GSE3456, GSE3812, GSE4398. Users can refer to the chapter "Microarray data analysis for transcriptome profiling" to get these data from GEO.

2.3 MATLAB Toolbox

MATLAB is a multiparadigm programming language which is intended primarily for numerical computing (https://www.mathworks.com/). It is a proprietary product of The MathWorks Inc., so users need to buy the license to use it. MATLAB has a vast library of prebuilt toolboxes that are designed for machine learning, signal processing, image processing, etc. Each toolbox could be purchased and loaded separately. In this protocol, we need the base of MATLAB, the LIBSVM library, and the mRMR library. The details of installing LIBSVM and mRMR will be introduced in their corresponding sections.

3 Methods

3.1 Data Processing and Loading

The downloaded gene expression noise data and all the expression data were compiled together as a single ASCII text file according to their gene names using custom Perl script. After that, the merged file could be loaded to MATLAB through different functions such as "importdata()" and "textscan()". It could also be loaded to MATLAB through GUI "Import Data" icon. Here, we show an example of using the function "importdata()":

```
GeneExpNoiseVar = importdata('GeneExpNoise.Var.txt');
```

where "GeneExpNoise.Var.txt" is the compiled ASCII text file and the returned variable *"GeneExpNoiseVar"* is a structure array. It includes two elements: "textdata" contains gene names and header, and "data" contains numerical array of gene expression noise and all the other gene expression profiles. For example, assume the first column of the "data" matrix is gene expression noise and the rest are the gene expression profile at different conditions, then we could get:

```
geneexpnoise = GeneExpNoiseVar.data(:,1);
geneexpvariations = GeneExpNoiseVar.data(:,2:end);
```

3.2 Examine Descriptive Statistics

1. To investigate the relationship between gene expression variation and noise, the natural choice is to first examine their correlation, which could be calculated using the MATLAB function corr(). In MATLAB console, type:

```
ρ = corr(geneexpnoise, geneexpvariations, 'type', 'Pearson', 'rows', 'pairwise');
```

where *"geneexpvariations"* could be any types of gene expression variations mentioned above.

2. After obtaining the correlations (here assume "CoRRArray" save the correlation results), users could visualize them by displaying the correlations into a figure (Fig. 1) using the following commands:

```
CoRRArrayLabels = {
'Response to various conditions';
'Stress response';
'Transcription plasticity';
'Mutation/knockout of chromatin regulators';
'Knockout of transcription factors';
'Variability among mutation accumulation lines';
'Variability among strain RM11-1a';
'Variability among strain BY4716';
'Variability between RM11-1a and BY4716';
'Variability between S288c and YKM789';
'Variability among 4 yeast species';
'Variability between 2 yeast species'
};
% Change the Y axis tick labels to use the CoRRArrayLabels
figure
barh(CoRRArray)
xlabel('Pearson correlation');
set(gca, 'YTick', 1:12);
set(gca, 'YTickLabel', CoRRArrayLabels);
```

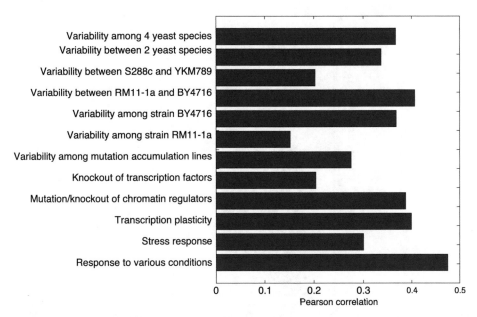

Fig. 1 Correlations between gene expression noise level and gene expression variations under different conditions. Each bar represents the Pearson correlation coefficient between noise level and expression variation obtained from respective conditions

3. Furthermore, it is also a good choice to visualize the correlation between noise level and expression variations, which could be performed using the function "scatter" in MATLAB. For example, type

```
scatter(geneexpnoise, geneexpvariations, 20,'b','filled')
xlabel('Measured DM')
ylabel('Response to various conditions')
```

It will show scatterplot between gene expression noise ("DM value") and gene expression variations under "response to various conditions" (a case in Fig. 1, Pearson correlation coefficient = 0.475) in filled dots with blue color (Fig. 2). Users could apply the same command to visualize the correlation for other conditions.

3.3 Support Vector Regression

Support vector regression (SVR) is a machine-learning algorithm to fit the regression problem. It is an extension of Support vector machine (SVM) which was initially introduced for solving classification problem in the early 1990s [35, 37, 38] (*see* **Note 1**). By implementing the maximum-margin principle, an ε-insensitive loss function is introduced to SVR where at most ε deviation is allowed from the actually obtained targets and at the same time requiring the regression function as flat as possible. When dealing with nonlinear regression, the feature vectors are first projected into a high

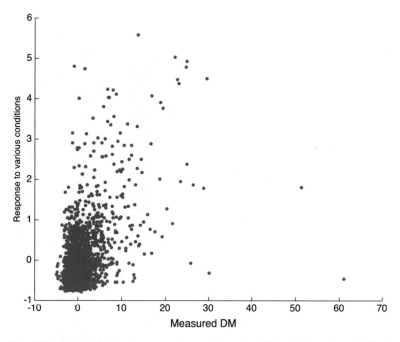

Fig. 2 Scatterplot between gene expression noise (DM value) and normalized gene expression variation under "response to various conditions". x-Axis represents the measured gene expression noise DM value while y-axis represents the normalized gene expression variation under "response to various conditions". This scatterplot was made based on 2050 genes that have both DM value and gene expression variation values

dimensional feature space with a kernel function, such as a Gaussian kernel: $K(x_i, x_j) = \exp \{- \parallel x_i - x_j \parallel^2 / 2\sigma^2\}$, and then the linear SVR procedure is applied in the high dimensional feature space. Please check details from [34, 39].

3.3.1 LIBSVM Installation

LIBSVM is a popular library which implements various types of SVM and SVR models. It is originally written in C++, but also with the interface to other programming languages and environments (e.g., R, MATLAB and Java) be provided.

In this protocol, we use the MATLAB interface of LIBSVM, which could be downloaded from LIBSVM website http://www.csie.ntu.edu.tw/~cjlin/libsvm/ (*see* **Note 2**). After downloading and uncompressing the package, the MATLAB implement could be found in the matlab subfolder. Change the working directory to that folder (e.g., /dir/for/libsvm), and then use the "make" command to compile it (*see* **Notes 3** and **4**):

```
cd /dir/for/libsvm
make
```

3.3.2 Data Scaling	We define gene expression variation data as input matrix (noted as "*geneexpvariations*") and gene expression noise data as real-valued training label data (noted as "*geneexpnoise*"). It is recommended to scale all the real-valued data into $[0,1]$ or $[-1,1]$. Here we scale both data into $[-1,1]$ by using the following command:

```
geneexpvar_data = geneexpvariations;
geneexpvar_data_scale = 2*( geneexpvar_data - repmat(min(geneexpvar_data,[],1),
size(geneexpvar_data,1),1)) * spdiags(1./(max(geneexpvar_data,[],1) -
min(geneexpvar_data,[],1))', 0, size(geneexpvar_data,2), size(geneexpvar_data,2)) -
ones(size(geneexpvar_data,1), size(geneexpvar_data,2));
geneexpnoise_scale = 2*(geneexpnoise - min(geneexpnoise)) / (max(geneexpnoise) -
min(geneexpnoise)) -1;
```

3.3.3 SVR Model Training	Once the MATLAB implement of LIBSVM is installed, we can build the SVR model and use the model to predict testing data. To train a SVR model, type:

```
SVRmodel = svmtrain(geneexpnoise_scale, geneexpvar_data_scale, 'libsvm_options');
```

where "*libsvm_options*" is the option setting for SVM models. In this protocol, we introduced the ε-SVR model with Gaussian kernel which corresponds to set "-s 3 -t 2". For the Gaussian kernel based ε-SVR model, there are hyperparameters such as regularization parameter "C", "σ" in the kernel function, and "ε". We will introduce how to select them in the following section.

3.3.4 SVR Model Prediction	After building the optimal SVR model ("*SVRmodel*"), we could use it to predict new testing data ("*geneexpvar_data_scale_tst*") with associated "*geneexpnoise_scale_tst*", type:

```
geneexpnoise_scale_tst_predict = svmpredict(geneexpnoise_scale_tst
geneexpvar_data_scale_tst, SVRmodel);
```

where "*geneexpnoise_scale_tst*" could be known value if running cross-validation (will mention it in Subheading 3.3.6), or could be any value if for predicting unknown testing data.

3.3.5 Performance Measurement	We used Pearson's correlation coefficient as the measurement to assess the performance of the regression model (*see* **Note 5**). Assume "*geneexpnoise_scale_tst*" is the real-value label vector after scaling, and "*geneexpnoise_scale_tst_predict*" is the predicted value from the SVR model, the correlation "ρ" could be calculated in MATLAB by typing:

```
ρ = corr(geneexpnoise_scale_tst,geneexpnoise_scale_tst_predict,'type','Pearson','rows',
'pairwise');
```

Whenever a classification needs to be assessed, the area under ROC (receiver operating characteristic) curve (AUC) was adopted. Many packages provide the ROC analysis in MATLAB. Here we introduce the function "perfcurve" embedded in MATLAB. We separate gene set into two classes: "noisy" (DM value ≥ 1) and "quiet" (DM value <1). We use the predicted value from the SVR model ("*geneexpnoise_scale_tst_predict*") as the score and compared with the given true class labels ("*noise_labels*" compiled with "noisy" and "quiet" array). In MATLAB, type:

```
[FPR, TPR, Thres, SVRAUC] = perfcurve(noise_labels, geneexpnoise_scale_tst_predict,
'noisy')
```

The returned variable "*SVRAUC*" gives the AUC score for the SVR score performance. We can also use "*plot(FPR, TPR)*" to generate the ROC curve.

3.3.6 Cross-Validation and Model Selection

Up to now, we introduced how to train a SVR model and make prediction using the model. The ultimate goal is to train a model that has robust performance on unknown testing data. If we use the whole available dataset to train a model, it may lead to overfitting [40, 41] which usually show worse performance on unknown testing data. One strategy is to simulate the procedure of predicting unknown data from a train model by using the so-called K-fold cross-validation strategy. That is, we randomly divided the whole gene sets into K disjoint sets of equal size. For each run, $K - 1$ folds of them are used as training dataset and the remaining one as the testing dataset. This process is then repeated K times with each of the K sets used exactly once as the validation data (*see* **Note 6**). Based on the K-fold cross-validation strategy, we then could use a grid search approach to select the optimal parameters. In this protocol we chose $K = 10$. In MATLAB, the tenfold cross-validation of input matrix and label data could be implemented by randomly generating indices of tenfold of the whole data set using the function "*crossvalind*". The process of tenfold cross-validation then could be coded as following:

```
function RHO = crossvalindperformance (geneexpnoise_scale, geneexpvar_data_scale,
K, 'libsvm_options')

indices = crossvalind( 'Kfold', [ geneexpnoise_scale geneexpvar_data_scale] , K);
% Based on the splitted 10-fold sets, we could perform the cross-validation process.
for i=1:K

Indextst = (indices ==i);
 Indextrn = ~Indextst;
  geneexpvar_data_scale_tst = geneexpvar_data_scale (Indextst,:);
 geneexpnoise_scale_tst = geneexpnoise_scale (Indextst,:);
 geneexpvar_data_scale_trn = geneexpvar_data_scale (Indextrn,:);
 geneexpnoise_scale_trn = geneexpnoise_scale (Indextrn,:);
```

```
SVRmodel = svmtrain(geneexpnoise_scale_trn, geneexpvar_data_scale_trn,
'libsvm_options');
      %train a SVR model
    [geneexpnoise_scale_tst_predict] = svmpredict(geneexpnoise_scale_tst,
geneexpvar_data_scale_tst,
 SVRmodel);

 % predict the output of geneexpvar_data_scale_tst using SVRmodel
 geneexpnoise_scale_predict(Indextst) = geneexpnoise_scale_tst_predict;
 end

RHO = corr(geneexpnoise_scale, geneexpnoise_scale_predict, 'type', 'Pearson');
% return the correlation between true real-value 'geneexpnoise_scale' and the
predicted
% 'geneexpnoise_scale_predict'.
end
```

Once we have the above "*crossvalindperformance*", we could use the grid search strategy to get the optimal hyper-parameters.

```
function [BestRHO,Ypredict, bestc, bestg, bestp ] = SVRtrain_grid(geneexpnoise_scale,
geneexpvar_data_scale, K, Cbegin, Cend, Cstep, Gbegin, Gend, Gstep, Pbegin, Pend,
Pstep)
    BestRHO=0;
   i = 1;
   for Cloop = Cbegin : Cstep : Cend
             c = 2^Cloop;
     for Gloop = Gbegin : Gstep : Gend
     g = 2^Gloop;
     for Ploop = Pbegin : Pstep : Pend
 p = 2^Ploop;
 C(i,1) = c;
 G(i,1) = g;
 P(i,1) = p;
 i = i + 1;
            end
          end
    end

   n=length(C);
       N=randperm(n)'; % randomly train SVR using different parameters.

   for j=1:n
 libsvm_options=[ ' -s 3 -t 2 -c ', num2str(C(N(j))),' -g ', num2str(G(N
(j))), ' -p ',
 num2str(P(N(j)))];
 % disp(sprintf('[Local] c=%f, g=%f, p =%f: ', C(N(j)), G(N(j)), P(N(j))));
 RHO = crossvalindperformance (geneexpnoise_scale, geneexpvar_data_scale, K,
 'libsvm_options')
 if (BestRHO <= RHO),
  BestRHO = RHO; bestc = C(N(j)); bestg = G(N(j)); bestp = P(N(j));
    end
 end
```

We have now obtained the optimal parameters for the SVR model (*see* **Note 7**).

3.4 Feature Selection

One of the important processes in machine learning is to find the most useful or most relevant features for prediction. This is a process called feature selection which generally could give a better predictive model or provide a better understanding of which features contribute to the predictive model. The feature selection algorithms are mainly separated into three categories [42]: (1) filter strategy—extracting features regardless of the model; (2) wrapper strategy—extracting a combination of informative features with a learning algorithm; (3) embedded strategy—performing feature selection and classification simultaneously. Filter strategies are widely used as it is computationally efficient. However, most of them do not consider the dependency between features and tend to select redundant features. Here we introduce a Mutual information based minimum redundancy–maximum relevance (mRMR) feature selection method [42–45] which selects features that have the highest relevance with the target classes and are also minimally redundant, i.e., features that are maximally dissimilar to each other. Briefly, given $I(f_i, y)$ represents the mutation information between the feature i and the class label y, the maximum-relevance method selects the top m features in the descent order of $I(f_i, y)$, i.e., the best m individual features correlated to the target class: $\max_s D = \frac{1}{|S|} \sum_{f_i \in S} I(f_i, y)$, where S denotes the subset of the features we are seeking. The minimum-redundancy method in another hand removes the redundance among features using: $\min_s R = \frac{1}{|S|^2} \sum_{f_i, f_j \in S} I(f_i, f_j)$. The minimum redundancy–maximum relevance (mRMR) feature selection selects the m-th feature from the set $\{F - S_{m-1}\}$ by maximizing $\max_{f_i \in F - Sm-1}[D - R]$, where F represents the set of features and S_{m-1} represents the already selected $m - 1$ features. This method has been successfully used for gene subset selection from microarray gene expression data [43]. For more details, please refer to the paper [45].

Although mRMR could handle both categorical and continuous variables, empirically the categorical one leads to better results than continuous one. Therefore, we simply binarize the real-value noise level into two classes ("noisy" and "quiet") based on whether DM $\geq$ 1 or not.

1. mRMR installation. The mRMR software is available from the website (http://home.penglab.com/proj/mRMR/) where both online version and offline version with different programming languages are available. In this protocol, we introduce the

MATLAB version of mRMR. From the website, clicking the MATLAB version of mRMR will link to MATLAB "File Exchange." To download the files from "File Exchange" of MATLAB, users first need to create an account from MATLAB and then login. To install MATLAB version of mRMR, users need to

(a) Install Mutual Information Computation toolbox provided by the same author, which could also be found at the website http://home.penglab.com/proj/mRMR/.

(b) From MATLAB, go to the working path, run list = dir('*.cpp'); to get the list of files.

(c) For all the files in list, change log(2) to log(2.0) if exists.

(d) Run "makeosmex.m" to compile the C++ source codes (*see* **Note 4**).

(e) Select the working folder, right click and select "Add to Path" to add the working path to MATLAB path.

2. Once the MATLAB packages are downloaded and installed correctly, we can perform the mRMR feature selection. It requires the class label variable, the data matrix of input features and the number of features to be selected. In MATLAB, type:

```
features = mrmr_miq_d(data, y, m)
```

where *data* is the input feature matrix, *y* is the class label, and *m* is the number of features need to be selected.

3. Given any of the selected features, the previous process of training SVR models is repeated and the cross-validation performance is reported. In this way, we could investigate which features have the highest predictive power and how many features may be sufficient to obtain decent predictive power. Particularly, using all 633 gene expression variation features as input for the SVR model and by separating genes into "noisy" and "quiet" sets (based on whether or not $DM \geq 1$), the ROC curve under tenfold cross-validation is shown in Fig. 3.

4. After applying the mRMR approach, we could calculate the performance of SVR using incremental top features (assume the results is saved in MATLAB as variable "SVRperf_topfeatures"). It could be visualized in Fig. 4 (up to $m = 40$ top features) using the following command:

```
plot(SVRperf_topfeatures,'LineWidth',6)
xlabel('Number of the top features');
ylabel('AUC scores');
```

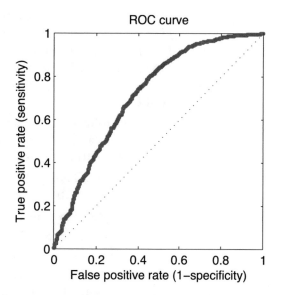

Fig. 3 ROC curve generated using tenfold cross-validation. ROC curve is generated from the modeled noise values by SVR and the corresponded AUC score is 0.72. The diagonal dash line represents the ROC curve from randomly guessing

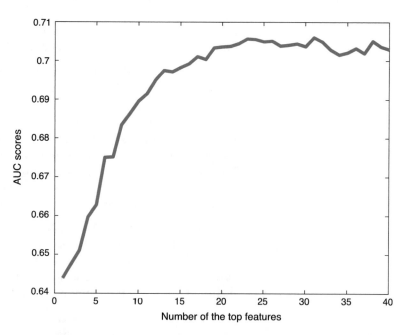

Fig. 4 Performance of the SVR model with incremental top m features. The selected top 20 features by mRMR method contribute mainly to the discrimination ability

From Fig. 4, it indicated that not all features are equally important and the discrimination performance of the SVR model saturated after top 20 features were used (the AUC score = 0.71).

3.5 Downstream Analysis

In term of ascertaining the predictive power of a valid regression model, appropriate validations are recommended. In this protocol, we introduce the validations of the predictive model by calculating the enrichment of noisy genes (or quiet genes) on different types of biological aspects such as dosage sensitivity and essentiality, hub genes in protein-protein interaction, as well as nucleosome positioning in promoter regions. In addition, we also validate the model by performing the prediction in other single-cell organisms (*see* **Note 8**).

In the dataset we used, 3909 of the genes do not have the measured noise level. We thus used the SVR model to obtain predicted noise level for these genes. As the true gene expression noise levels for these genes are not available, we cannot validate the SVR prediction directly. Therefore, we sought to use other features to validate it in an indirect way. We first divided these 3909 genes into two groups: "noisy" genes (1844 genes with DM $\geq$ 1) and "quiet" genes (2065 genes with DM $<$ 1). Then, we investigate whether or not the predicted noisy genes show enrichment on haploinsufficient genes or essential genes. We observed a higher number of haploinsufficient genes and essential genes in quiet genes than noisy genes (Wilcoxon rank sum test, $P = 1.2e-5$ and $P = 4.1e-3$ for haploinsufficient genes and essential genes, respectively). We also observed that hub proteins in protein-protein interaction networks are highly enriched in "quiet" genes (Wilcoxon rank sum test, $P = 4.2e-4$), which is consistent with the fact that "quiet" genes are more conserved than "noisy" genes at the sequence level [12, 46, 47]. Recent measured nucleosome positioning data [48] also provide us another view to validate the predicted noisy gene set. Specifically, it is documented that variably expressed genes tend to possess nucleosome in the promoter regions [49]. We thus used the available nucleosome positioning data to calculate the mean occupancy for different genes, and found that the measured and predicted noisier genes (genes with top 5% of predicted and measured DM values) had significantly higher nucleosome occupancy than other genes, i.e., their promoters are in a more "closed state" (Wilcoxon rank sum test, $P = 2.3e-5$ for measured noisier genes, and $P = 3.8e-4$ for modeled noisier genes, respectively) [39].

4   Notes

1. Support vector machines or support vector regressions belong to a class of machine learning algorithms, which could avoid

"curse of dimensionality" (overfitting) even when the sample size is small. In other words, it is suitable for dataset with the so-called "large p, small m" problem (where p is the number of features and m is the number of samples), which are the cases in many bioinformatics problems such as gene expression data, SNP array data, etc.

2. MATLAB provides "Support Vector Machine Regression" module in the Statistics and Machine Learning Toolbox™, which is different from the MATLAB version of LIBSVM. Please check http://www.csie.ntu.edu.tw/~cjlin/libsvm/ for details.

3. If make.m does not work on MATLAB, then you need to type "mex -setup" to rebuild the package where a suitable compiler needs to be provided for mex. After that, you may rerun "make" again.

4. MATLAB provides the interface to call functions and subroutines written in the programming languages C/C++, Fortran, Python, etc. The wrapped functions are compiled and termed as "MEX-files". When installing (via "mex" function) "LIBSVM" or "Mutual Information Computation toolbox," users need to ensure there is a proper complier for C++ in their system environments.

5. A common way to measure the error for a regression model is to calculate the mean squared error (MSE) or the root mean squared error (RMSE). But for some specific purpose, the Pearson correlation or the Spearman correlation measurement are also used for assessing the performance.

6. In terms of cross-validation, to date, another popular way is to pick a small proportion of the whole dataset as an independent testing data, and then perform the cross-validation testing on the remaining ones.

7. Usually, less complex model would give more generalized ability. If achieving similar accuracy between two models when performing cross-validation, the model with smaller number of support vectors is preferred. For more detailed information about SVM, SVR and their extensions using LIBSVM, please refer to [36] and http://www.csie.ntu.edu.tw/~cjlin/libsvm/.

8. We demonstrated the relationship between gene expression variations and noise in single-cell organisms. It would be possible to extend it to multicellular organisms attribute to the rapidly developed single-cell sequencing techniques.

References

1. Raser JM, O'Shea EK (2005) Noise in gene expression: origins, consequences, and control. Science 309(5743):2010–2013. https://doi.org/10.1126/science.1105891

2. Basehoar AD, Zanton SJ, Pugh BF (2004) Identification and distinct regulation of yeast TATA box-containing genes. Cell 116 (5):699–709

3. Rao CV, Wolf DM, Arkin AP (2002) Control, exploitation and tolerance of intracellular noise. Nature 420(6912):231–237. https://doi.org/10.1038/nature01258

4. Kaern M, Elston TC, Blake WJ, Collins JJ (2005) Stochasticity in gene expression: from theories to phenotypes. Nat Rev Genet 6 (6):451–464. https://doi.org/10.1038/nrg1615

5. Karmakar R, Bose I (2004) Graded and binary responses in stochastic gene expression. Phys Biol 1(3-4):197–204. https://doi.org/10.1088/1478-3967/1/4/001

6. Brem RB, Kruglyak L (2005) The landscape of genetic complexity across 5,700 gene expression traits in yeast. Proc Natl Acad Sci U S A 102(5):1572–1577. https://doi.org/10.1073/pnas.0408709102

7. Brem RB, Yvert G, Clinton R, Kruglyak L (2002) Genetic dissection of transcriptional regulation in budding yeast. Science 296 (5568):752–755. https://doi.org/10.1126/science.1069516

8. Townsend JP, Cavalieri D, Hartl DL (2003) Population genetic variation in genome-wide gene expression. Mol Biol Evol 20 (6):955–963. https://doi.org/10.1093/molbev/msg106

9. Tirosh I, Weinberger A, Bezalel D, Kaganovich M, Barkai N (2008) On the relation between promoter divergence and gene expression evolution. Mol Syst Biol 4:159. https://doi.org/10.1038/msb4100198

10. Wolf L, Silander OK, van Nimwegen E (2015) Expression noise facilitates the evolution of gene regulation. Elife 4. https://doi.org/10.7554/eLife.05856

11. Charlebois DA (2015) Effect and evolution of gene expression noise on the fitness landscape. Phys Rev E 92(2):022713. https://doi.org/10.1103/PhysRevE.92.022713

12. Lehner B (2008) Selection to minimise noise in living systems and its implications for the evolution of gene expression. Mol Syst Biol 4:170. https://doi.org/10.1038/msb.2008.11

13. Zhang Z, Qian W, Zhang J (2009) Positive selection for elevated gene expression noise in yeast. Mol Syst Biol 5:299. https://doi.org/10.1038/msb.2009.58

14. Elowitz MB, Levine AJ, Siggia ED, Swain PS (2002) Stochastic gene expression in a single cell. Science 297(5584):1183–1186. https://doi.org/10.1126/science.1070919

15. Becskei A, Serrano L (2000) Engineering stability in gene networks by autoregulation. Nature 405(6786):590–593. https://doi.org/10.1038/35014651

16. Pedraza JM, van Oudenaarden A (2005) Noise propagation in gene networks. Science 307 (5717):1965–1969. https://doi.org/10.1126/science.1109090

17. Newman JR, Ghaemmaghami S, Ihmels J, Breslow DK, Noble M, DeRisi JL, Weissman JS (2006) Single-cell proteomic analysis of S. cerevisiae reveals the architecture of biological noise. Nature 441(7095):840–846. https://doi.org/10.1038/nature04785

18. Colman-Lerner A, Gordon A, Serra E, Chin T, Resnekov O, Endy D, Pesce CG, Brent R (2005) Regulated cell-to-cell variation in a cell-fate decision system. Nature 437 (7059):699–706. https://doi.org/10.1038/nature03998

19. Sanchez A, Golding I (2013) Genetic determinants and cellular constraints in noisy gene expression. Science 342(6163):1188–1193. https://doi.org/10.1126/science.1242975

20. Paulsson J (2004) Summing up the noise in gene networks. Nature 427(6973):415–418. https://doi.org/10.1038/nature02257

21. Kumar N, Platini T, Kulkarni RV (2014) Exact distributions for stochastic gene expression models with bursting and feedback. Phys Rev Lett 113(26):268105. https://doi.org/10.1103/PhysRevLett.113.268105

22. Singh A, Soltani M (2013) Quantifying intrinsic and extrinsic variability in stochastic gene expression models. PLoS One 8(12):e84301. https://doi.org/10.1371/journal.pone.0084301

23. Paulsson J (2005) Models of stochastic gene expression. Phys Life Rev 2(2):157–175. https://doi.org/10.1016/j.plrev.2005.03.003

24. Sanchez A, Kondev J (2008) Transcriptional control of noise in gene expression. Proc Natl Acad Sci U S A 105(13):5081–5086. https://doi.org/10.1073/pnas.0707904105

25. Zheng XD, Tao Y (2011) Stochastic analysis of gene expression. Methods Mol Biol 734:123–151. https://doi.org/10.1007/978-1-61779-086-7_7

26. Gui R, Liu Q, Yao Y, Deng H, Ma C, Jia Y, Yi M (2016) Noise decomposition principle in a coherent feed-forward transcriptional regulatory loop. Front Physiol 7:600. https://doi.org/10.3389/fphys.2016.00600

27. Ihmels J, Friedlander G, Bergmann S, Sarig O, Ziv Y, Barkai N (2002) Revealing modular organization in the yeast transcriptional

network. Nat Genet 31(4):370–377. https://doi.org/10.1038/ng941

28. Tirosh I, Barkai N (2008) Two strategies for gene regulation by promoter nucleosomes. Genome Res 18(7):1084–1091. https://doi.org/10.1101/gr.076059.108

29. Gasch AP, Spellman PT, Kao CM, Carmel-Harel O, Eisen MB, Storz G, Botstein D, Brown PO (2000) Genomic expression programs in the response of yeast cells to environmental changes. Mol Biol Cell 11 (12):4241–4257

30. Landry CR, Lemos B, Rifkin SA, Dickinson WJ, Hartl DL (2007) Genetic properties influencing the evolvability of gene expression. Science 317(5834):118–121. https://doi.org/10.1126/science.1140247

31. Gagneur J, Sinha H, Perocchi F, Bourgon R, Huber W, Steinmetz LM (2009) Genome-wide allele- and strand-specific expression profiling. Mol Syst Biol 5:274. https://doi.org/10.1038/msb.2009.31

32. Steinfeld I, Shamir R, Kupiec M (2007) A genome-wide analysis in Saccharomyces cerevisiae demonstrates the influence of chromatin modifiers on transcription. Nat Genet 39 (3):303–309. https://doi.org/10.1038/ng1965

33. Hu Z, Killion PJ, Iyer VR (2007) Genetic reconstruction of a functional transcriptional regulatory network. Nat Genet 39 (5):683–687. https://doi.org/10.1038/ng2012

34. Smola AJ, Scholkopf B (2004) A tutorial on support vector regression. Stat Comput 14 (3):199–222. https://doi.org/10.1023/B:Stco.0000035301.49549.88

35. Deng N, Tian Y, Zhang C (2012) Support vector machines: optimization based theory, algorithms, and extensions. Chapman and Hall/CRC, London

36. Chang CC, Lin CJ (2011) LIBSVM: a library for support vector machines. ACM T Intel Syst Tec 2(3). https://doi.org/10.1145/1961189.1961199

37. Vapnik VN (1995) The nature of statistical learning theory. Springer, New York, NY

38. Guyon I, Weston J, Barnhill S, Vapnik V (2002) Gene selection for cancer classification using support vector machines. Mach Learn 46 (1-3):389–422. https://doi.org/10.1023/A:1012487302797

39. Dong D, Shao X, Deng N, Zhang Z (2011) Gene expression variations are predictive for stochastic noise. Nucleic Acids Res 39 (2):403–413. https://doi.org/10.1093/nar/gkq844

40. Hawkins DM (2004) The problem of overfitting. J Chem Inf Comput Sci 44(1):1–12. https://doi.org/10.1021/ci0342472

41. Tetko IV, Livingstone DJ, Luik AI (1995) Neural-network studies. 1. Comparison of overfitting and overtraining. J Chem Inf Comput Sci 35(5):826–833. https://doi.org/10.1021/Ci00027a006

42. Hira ZM, Gillies DF (2015) A review of feature selection and feature extraction methods applied on microarray data. Adv Bioinformatics 2015:198363. https://doi.org/10.1155/2015/198363

43. Zhang Y, Ding C, Li T (2008) Gene selection algorithm by combining reliefF and mRMR. BMC Genomics 9(Suppl 2):S27. https://doi.org/10.1186/1471-2164-9-S2-S27

44. Ding C, Peng H (2005) Minimum redundancy feature selection from microarray gene expression data. J Bioinform Comput Biol 3 (2):185–205

45. Peng H, Long F, Ding C (2005) Feature selection based on mutual information: criteria of max-dependency, max-relevance, and min-redundancy. IEEE Trans Pattern Anal Mach Intell 27(8):1226–1238. https://doi.org/10.1109/TPAMI.2005.159

46. Li J, Min R, Vizeacoumar FJ, Jin K, Xin X, Zhang Z (2010) Exploiting the determinants of stochastic gene expression in Saccharomyces cerevisiae for genome-wide prediction of expression noise. Proc Natl Acad Sci U S A 107(23):10472–10477. https://doi.org/10.1073/pnas.0914302107

47. Raj A, van Oudenaarden A (2008) Nature, nurture, or chance: stochastic gene expression and its consequences. Cell 135(2):216–226. https://doi.org/10.1016/j.cell.2008.09.050

48. Kaplan N, Moore IK, Fondufe-Mittendorf Y, Gossett AJ, Tillo D, Field Y, LeProust EM, Hughes TR, Lieb JD, Widom J, Segal E (2009) The DNA-encoded nucleosome organization of a eukaryotic genome. Nature 458 (7236):362–366. https://doi.org/10.1038/nature07667

49. Choi JK, Kim YJ (2009) Intrinsic variability of gene expression encoded in nucleosome positioning sequences. Nat Genet 41(4):498–503. https://doi.org/10.1038/ng.319

Chapter 14

A Protocol for Epigenetic Imprinting Analysis with RNA-Seq Data

Jinfeng Zou, Daoquan Xiang, Raju Datla, and Edwin Wang

Abstract

Genomic imprinting is an epigenetic regulatory mechanism that operates through expression of certain genes from maternal or paternal in a parent-of-origin-specific manner. Imprinted genes have been identified in diverse biological systems that are implicated in some human diseases and in embryonic and seed developmental programs in plants. The molecular underpinning programs and mechanisms involved in imprinting are yet to be explored in depth in plants. The recent advances in RNA-Seq-based methods and technologies offer an opportunity to systematically analyze epigenetic imprinting that operates at the whole genome level in the model and crop plants. We are interested using Arabidopsis model system, to investigate gene expression patterns associated with parent of origin and their implications to imprinting during embryo and seed development. Toward this, we have generated early embryo development RNA-Seq-based transcriptome datasets in F1s from a genetic cross between two diverse Arabidopsis thaliana ecotypes Col-0 and Tsu-1. With the data, we developed a protocol for evaluating the maternal and paternal contributions of genes during the early stages of embryo development after fertilization. This protocol is also designed to consider the contamination from other potential seed tissues, sequencing quality, proper processing of sequenced reads and variant calling, and appropriate inference of the parental contributions based on the parent-of-origin-specific single-nucleotide polymorphisms within the expressed genes. The approach, methods and the protocol developed in this study can be used for evaluating the effects of epigenetic imprinting in plants.

Key words Genomic imprinting, RNA-Seq, Maternal and paternal contributions, *Arabidopsis thaliana*

1 Introduction

Genomic imprinting is a type of regulation by epigenetic inheritance. The allele inherited from the mother or the father could be imprinted which involve silencing of that allele with potential effects on the offspring. The well-known example for imprinting is the findings from the cross between donkey and horse: a hinny is produced by a male horse and a female donkey whereas a mule by a female horse and a male donkey [1]. Studies also showed that the imprinting plays important roles in diseases like obesity and

Yejun Wang and Ming-an Sun (eds.), *Transcriptome Data Analysis: Methods and Protocols*, Methods in Molecular Biology, vol. 1751, https://doi.org/10.1007/978-1-4939-7710-9_14, © Springer Science+Business Media, LLC 2018

psychiatric disorders [2]. In the model plant Arabidopsis, a phenotype of low seed weight is shown by inheriting extramaternal genomes while the reciprocal phenotype of high seed weight with extrapaternal genomes [3].

In sexually reproducing organisms, fertilization of an egg and a sperm produces zygote. In most mammals, the zygote genome is transcriptionally quiescent after fertilization but is activated after several rounds of cell divisions and also the early embryogenesis depends on the maternally inherited transcripts from the egg cell [4, 5]. It has been shown that after the activation of the zygote genome, with the progressive degradation of the maternal transcripts, the expression program gradually switches to biparental transcripts ensuing the control of the subsequent development [4, 5]. The duration of maternal control before the activation of zygotic genome varies in different species from 1 to 15 cell cycles [4]. In flowering plants, the length of this duration and how the parental contribution is regulated and specified are not very clear. In the model plant Arabidopsis, only few studies have focused on this but targeted only few genes [6, 7]. Recently, the RNA-Seq-based transcriptome studies were conducted on this issue in Arabidopsis [4, 8, 9]. However, the findings are not consistent and inconclusive. Nodine et al. reported equal contributions of maternal and paternal genomes [9], while Autran et al. showed maternal dominance [4]. Recently, Del Toro-De Leó et al. reconciled the contradiction by reporting the nonequivalent contributions of parental genomes with significant number of maternally expressed genes essential for embryo development [8].

The inconsistency among independent studies could be attributed to preparation of pure samples caused by the contamination with other tissues, low-quality sequencing of transcripts, and improper process of sequenced reads, incorrect variant calling and inappropriate analyses. A major bottleneck to investigate molecular aspects of early embryogenesis in plants is the access to early embryo stages. We developed methods for isolating single-cell zygotes in Arabidopsis, as well as other representative stages of early embryo development including zygote, octant, globular along with later stages of heart, torpedo, bent and mature embryos in the model plant Arabidopsis [10]. To avoid and prevent mRNA contamination from the surrounding ovule tissues and endosperm, the isolated embryos were washed and the representative embryo stages were confirmed by observation under microscope. Here, we have elaborated the protocol that was developed based on the zygote stage RNA-Seq data. Next, the evaluation of maternal and paternal contributions for the early embryogenesis was performed firstly by preprocessing the raw RNA-Seq data, secondly by evaluating the contamination of other tissues, thirdly by identifying the maternal-/paternal-specific SNPs in the expressed genes. In order to assuring the reliability of the selected SNPs, those assigned with at least ten reads were considered for the analysis to assign expression from (a) maternal or (b) paternal or (c) both. Note that this enrichment and stringent process might reduce the coverage and capture of the true parent-of-origin-specific SNPs in the case of low read depth. Finally, the parental contributions were evaluated based on the ratio of the read counts for the maternal and paternal alleles.

2 Materials

2.1 Data

Arabidopsis thaliana ecotypes Col-0, Tsu-1 and their cross Col-0 × Tsu-1 (two biological replicates for each) were sequenced on Illumina HiSeq (pair-end). The unfertilized Col-0 ovule was also sequenced to evaluate the contamination of other tissues.

Arabidopsis reference genome and gene annotation files were downloaded from (http://plants.ensembl.org/Arabidopsis_thaliana/Info/Index).

2.2 Tools

A list of software tools are used for the imprinting analysis and shown below. They should be installed and configured according to the manuals or documents listed in corresponding websites.

1. Sickle (https://github.com/najoshi/sickle).
2. Bowtie 2 (https://sourceforge.net/projects/bowtie-bio/files/bowtie2/, version 2.2.3).
3. Htseq (https://github.com/simon-anders/htseq).
4. SAMtools (http://samtools.sourceforge.net, version 1.3.1).
5. Bamtools (https://sourceforge.net/projects/bamtools/, version 2.3.0).
6. Picard-tools (https://sourceforge.net/projects/picard/, version 1.103).
7. GenomeAnalysisTK (https://software.broadinstitute.org/gatk/download/, version 3.4-0).
8. R (https://www.r-project.org/, version 3.1.1).
9. edgeR (https://bioconductor.org/packages/release/bioc/html/edgeR.html).

3 Methods

3.1 Overall Pipeline of the Analysis

The pipeline can be divided into the following four major steps:

3.1.1 Alignment of Reads to the Reference Genome

The sequenced reads are required to be aligned to the reference genome. Before performing this step, the quality control for the raw reads has to be done. Because the sequenced reads usually have deteriorating quality toward the 3′-end and some toward the 5′-end as well, including these will negatively impact subsequent analyses. Therefore, Sickle was used to trim the 3′-end and/or 5′-end of reads or the whole reads according to the quality [11, 12]. Then, Bowtie 2 [13] was used to align the reads to the reference genome. This offers an ultrafast and memory-efficient tool for alignment, particularly good at aligning reads of about 50 up to 100s or 1000s of characters. Furthermore, Bowtie 2 supports gapped, local, and paired-end alignment modes.

3.1.2 Contamination Evaluation

Besides controlling the contamination of the surrounding tissues during the preparation of early stage embryo samples, an evaluation was also performed on the ovule tissue RNA-Seq data. This approach and comparative analysis was used to investigate differentially expressed genes between the unfertilized Col-0 ovule and the Col-0 × Tsu-1 zygote data. We believe that the more differentially expressed genes that are specific to embryo are selected and used, there will be less contamination and contribution of false positives for assigning maternally enriched transcripts.

3.1.3 SNP Calling

RNA sequencing technology measures the levels of mRNA transcripts. As many transcripts expected to derive from the alternative splicing mechanism, the reads may include parts of introns. This could especially influence the variant calling. To address this concern, the GATK tool of SplitNCigarReads was used, which is specifically designed to split the reads into exon segments (getting rid of Ns but maintaining grouping information) and hard-clip any sequences overhanging into the intronic regions. Then, the variant was called based on the processed reads.

3.1.4 Analysis of Maternal and Paternal Contributions

First, the maternal- and paternal-specific SNPs were selected by comparing the SNPs in the expressed genes of a cross while considering its parent separately. Then, the read counts of the parent-of-origin-specific SNPs and of the reference gene were summarized on gene level with the average values, in order to reduce the effect of sequencing issues (e.g., biases produced by the amplification procedure and low-mapping quality). The average read counts of the maternal- and paternal-specific SNPs are denoted as AvgSNPm and AvgSNPp, while the corresponding denotations for the reference gene are AvgREFm and AvgREFp. Second, for genes annotated with both maternal- and paternal-specific SNPs, the average read counts of the corresponding SNPs were used to calculate the parent-of-origin contributions as AvgSNPm/(AvgSNPm + AvgSNPp) for maternal contribution and AvgSNPp/(AvgSNPm + AvgSNPp) for paternal contribution. Third, for genes assigned with maternal- or paternal-specific SNPs, the average read counts of the reference genome could be derived from maternal and/or paternal contributions. We assumed that the contribution from the parent-of-origin with SNPs is equal to the average counts of the parent-of-origin-specific SNPs, or zero. Then, the average read counts from the reference gene were evaluated as AvgREFm = nAvgSNPm + AvgREFp for maternal-specific gene or AvgREFp = nAvgSNPp + AvgREFm for paternal-specific gene, n = 0 or 1. Then, the maternal and paternal contributions were estimated as AvgSNPm/(AvgSNPm + AvgREFp) and AvgREFp/(AvgSNPm + AvgREFp).

3.2 Align RNA-Seq Reads to the Reference Genome and Quantify the Corresponding Genes' Expression

In this protocol, TAIR 10 is used (http://www.arabidopsis.org).

1. Control the quality of pair-end reads.

```
$ sickle pe -t Illumina -f crossSeq_R1.fastq -r crossSeq_R2.
fastq -o
crossSeq_R1_trimmed.fastq -p crossSeq_R2_trimmed.fastq -s
crossSeq_singles_trimmed.fastq
```

2. Map the reads to the reference genome.

```
$ bowtie2 -p 16 -X 1500 -x refGenome.fa -1 crossSeq_R1_trimmed.
fastq -2 crossSeq _R2_trimmed.fastq -S crossSeq_trimmed.sam
--no-unal
```

3. Convert the sam file to bam file and sort the reads in the file.

```
$ samtools view -@ 8 -Sb crossSeq_trimmed.sam -o crossSeq_
trimmed.bam
$ samtools sort -@ 8 crossSeq_trimmed.bam crossSeq_trimmed_
sorted
$ samtools index crossSeq_sorted.bam
```

4. Count reads for genes.

```
$ htseq-count -m intersection-strict -s no -i gene_id --quiet
crossSeq_trimmed.sam geneAnnotation.gtf > crossSeq_counts.txt
```

3.3 Evaluate Contamination

1. Filter noise for read count.
   In R environment, run the following commands:

```
> raw <- read.csv('crossSeq_counts.txt', header=T, sep='\t')
> count.cross <- raw[, -1]
> row.names(count.cross) <- as.character(raw[,1])
> count.cross [count.cross <5] <- 0
```

The count profile for Col-0 ovule (count.parent) was also generated with the above script.

2. Identify differentially expressed genes
   R package 'edgeR' was used for gene expression comparison.

```
> library(edgeR)
> strain <- as.factor(c('cross', 'parent'))
> y <- DGEList(counts=cbind(count.cross, count.parent),
group= strain)
> y <- calcNormFactors(y)
> y <- estimateCommonDisp(y)
> y <- estimateTagwiseDisp(y)
> et <- exactTest(y, pair=unique(strain))
> et.g <- topTags(et, n=G)[[1]]
> deg <- et.g $FDR< 0.001 & abs(et.g $logFC)>=log2(2)
```

3.4 Call SNPs

SNPs were called with a combination of SAMtools, Bamtools, Picard-tools, and GenomeAnalysisTK.

1. Verify mate-pair information with picard-tools.

```
$ mkdir crossSeq_tmp
$ java -Djava.io.tmpdir=crossSeq_tmp -jar FixMateInformation.
jar
I=crossSeq_sorted.bam O=crossSeq_fxmt.bam SO=coordinate CRE-
ATE_INDEX=true
VALIDATION_STRINGENCY=SILENT
```

2. Filter out reads mapped improperly.

```
$ bamtools filter -isMapped true -isPaired true -isProperPair
true -in crossSeq_fxmt.bam -out crossSeq_fxmt_flt.bam
$ samtools index crossSeq_fxmt_flt.bam
```

3. Mark duplicate reads which are not counted for SNPs with Picard-tools.

```
$ java -jar MarkDuplicates.jar I=crossSeq_fxmt_flt.bam
O=crossSeq_fxmt_flt_dedupped.bam CREATE_INDEX=true
VALIDATION_STRINGENCY=SILENT M=output.metrics
```

4. Replace all read groups with a single new read group with Picard-tools.

```
$ java -jar AddOrReplaceReadGroups.jar I=crossSeq_fxmt_flt_
dedupped.bam
O=crossSeq_fxmt_flt_dedupped_added.bam SO=coordinate RGID=id
RGLB=library RGPL=platform RGPU=machine RGSM=sample
```

5. Remove reads with low mapping-quality.

```
$ bamtools filter -mapQuality ">=40" -in crossSeq_fxmt_flt_
dedupped_added.bam -out crossSeq_fxmt_flt_dedupped_
added_rmlq.bam
$ samtools index crossSeq_fxmt_flt_dedupped_added_rmlq.bam
```

6. Split reads into exon segments and hard-clip any sequences overhanging into the intronic regions

```
$ java -jar /home/ccb6/jinfeng/worknrc/tool/GenomeAnalysis
TK-3.4-0/GenomeAnalysisTK.jar -T SplitNCigarReads -R refGenome.
fa -I crossSeq_fxmt_flt_dedupped_added_rmlq.bam -o crossSeq_
split.bam -U ALLOW_N_CIGAR_READS
```

7. Recalibrate the quality score for every read with GenomeAnalysisTK.

```
$ java -Djava.io.tmpdir=crossSeq_tmp -jar GenomeAnalysisTK.jar
-T BaseRecalibrator -I crossSeq_split.bam -R refGenome.fa -o
crossSeq_recal_data.grp
$ java -Djava.io.tmpdir=crossSeq_tmp -jar GenomeAnalysisTK.jar
-T PrintReads -I crossSeq_split.bam -R refGenome.fa -o cross-
Seq_realigned_recal.bam -BQSR crossSeq-1_recal_data.grp
```

8. Call variants.

```
$ samtools mpileup -uf refGenome.fa crossSeq_split.bam |
bcftools view -vcg - > crossSeq.raw.0.bcf
$ bcftools view crossSeq.raw.0.bcf | vcfutils.pl varFilter
-D100 > crossSeq.raw.vcf
```

3.5 Select Parent-of-Origin-Specific SNPs

The maternal and paternal SNPs are produced with the above SNP calling procedure.

1. Filter SNPs with reads less than 10.

```
$ awk -F'DP4=' '{print $2}' maternal.raw.vcf | awk -F','
'{nSNP=$3+$4; if(nSNP>=10){print NR;}}' > maternal.nRow
$ awk 'NR==FNR{ pat [$0]; next} FNR in pat {print $0}'
maternal.nRow maternal.raw.vcf > maternal.flt.vcf
$ awk -F'DP4=' '{print $2}' paternal.raw.vcf | awk -F','
'{nSNP=$3+$4; if(nSNP>=10){print NR;}}' > paternal.nRow
$ awk 'NR==FNR{ pat [$0]; next} FNR in pat {print $0}'
paternal.nRow paternal.raw.vcf > paternal.flt.vcf
$ awk -F'DP4=' '{print $2}' crossSeq.raw.vcf | awk -F','
'{nSNP=$3+$4; if(nSNP>=10){print NR;}}' > crossSeq.nRow
$ awk 'NR==FNR{pat[$0]; next} FNR in pat {print $0}' crossSeq.
nRow crossSeq.raw.vcf > crossSeq.flt.vcf
```

2. Extract parent-of-origin-specific SNPs.

```
$ awk '{print $1"\t"$2"\t"$3"\t"$4"\t"$5}' maternal.flt.vcf |
sort > maternal.flt.1.vcf
$ awk '{print $1"\t"$2"\t"$3"\t"$4"\t"$5}' paternal.flt.vcf |
sort > paternal.flt.1.vcf
$ comm -3 maternal.flt.1.vcf paternal.flt.1.vcf > maternal.sp.
vcf
$ comm -3 paternal.flt.1.vcf maternal.flt.1.vcf > paternal.sp.
vcf
```

3. Select parent-of-origin SNPs in cross.

```
$ awk '{print $1"\t"$2"\t"$3"\t"$4"\t"$5}' crossSeq.flt.vcf >
crossSeq.flt.1.vcf
$ awk 'NR==FNR{pat[$0]; next} $0 in pat {print FNR}' maternal.
sp.vcf crossSeq.flt.1.vcf > crossSeq.maternal.sp.nRow
$ awk 'NR==FNR{pat[$0]; next} FNR in pat {print $0}' crossSeq.
maternal.sp.nRow crossSeq.flt.vcf > crossSeq.maternal.sp.vcf
$ awk 'NR==FNR{pat[$0]; next} $0 in pat {print FNR}' paternal.
sp.vcf crossSeq.flt.1.vcf > crossSeq.paternal.sp.nRow
$ awk 'NR==FNR{pat[$0]; next} FNR in pat {print $0}' crossSeq.
paternal.sp.nRow crossSeq.flt.vcf > crossSeq.paternal.sp.vcf
```

3.6 Output Parent-of-Origin-Specific Read Numbers in Gene Level

1. Extract the number of reads aligned to reference genome or with SNPs for parent-of-origin-specific SNPs

```
$ awk '{print $1}' crossSeq.maternal.sp.vcf > crossSeq.
maternal.sp.SNPgene
$ awk -F'DP4=' '{print $2}' crossSeq.maternal.sp.vcf | awk
-F',' '{nRef=$1+$2; nSNP=$3+$4; print nRef"\t"nSNP;}' >
crossSeq.maternal.sp.readCount
$ paste crossSeq.maternal.sp.SNPgene crossSeq.maternal.sp.
readCount > crossSeq.maternal.sp.SNP.ReadCount
$ awk '{print $1}' crossSeq.parental.sp.vcf > crossSeq.
parental.sp.SNPgene
$ awk -F'DP4=' '{print $2}' crossSeq.parental.sp.vcf | awk
-F',' '{nRef=$1+$2; nSNP=$3+$4; print $1"\t"nRef"\t"nSNP;}' >
crossSeq.parental.sp.readCount
$ paste crossSeq. parental.sp.SNPgene crossSeq.parental.sp.
readCount > crossSeq.parental.sp.SNP. ReadCount
```

2. Summarize the number of reads for parent-of-origin-specific SNPs in gene level with the average value

```
$ awk '{print $1}' crossSeq.maternal.sp.vcf | sort | uniq >
crossSeq.maternal.sp.gene
$ awk 'NR==FNR{sumRef[$0]=0; nRef[$0]=0; sumSNP[$0]=0; nSNP
[$0]=0; gene[FNR]=$0; next} $1 in sumRef {sumRef[$1]=sumRef
```

```
[$1]+$2; nRef[$1]=nRef[$1]+1; sumSNP[$1]=sumSNP[$1]+$3; nSNP
[$1]=nSNP[$1]+1;} END{for(i=1;i&lt;=(NR-FNR);i++){if(nRef
[gene[i]]==0){avgRef=0;}else{avgRef=sumRef[gene[i]]/nRef[gene
[i]]}; if(nSNP[gene[i]]==0){avgSNP=0;}else{avgSNP=sumSNP[gene
[i]]/nSNP[gene[i]]}; print avgRef"\t"avgSNP;}}' crossSeq.
maternal.sp.gene crossSeq.maternal.sp.SNP.ReadCount > cross-
Seq.maternal.sp.gene.ReadCount.0
$ paste crossSeq.maternal.sp.gene crossSeq.maternal.sp.gene.
ReadCount.0 > crossSeq.maternal.sp.gene.ReadCount
$ awk '{print $1}' crossSeq.paternal.sp.vcf | sort | uniq >
crossSeq. paternal.sp.gene
$ awk 'NR==FNR{sumRef[$0]=0; nRef[$0]=0; sumSNP[$0]=0; nSNP
[$0]=0; gene[FNR]=$0; next} $1 in sumRef {sumRef[$1]=sumRef
[$1]+$2; nRef[$1]=nRef[$1]+1; sumSNP[$1]=sumSNP[$1]+$3; nSNP
[$1]=nSNP[$1]+1;} END{for(i=1;i&lt;=(NR-FNR);i++){ if(nRef
[gene[i]]==0){avgRef=0;}else{avgRef=sumRef[gene[i]]/nRef[gene
[i]]}; if(nSNP[gene[i]]==0){avgSNP=0;}else{avgSNP=sumSNP[gene
[i]]/nSNP[gene[i]]}; print avgRef"\t"avgSNP;}}' crossSeq.
paternal.sp.gene crossSeq. paternal.sp.SNP.ReadCount >
crossSeq. paternal.sp.gene.ReadCount.0
$ paste crossSeq. paternal.sp.gene crossSeq. paternal.sp.gene.
ReadCount.0 > crossSeq. paternal.sp.gene.ReadCount
```

3.7 Calculate the Maternal and Paternal Contributions for Genes

1. Calculate the contributions for genes with both maternal- and paternal-specific SNPs

```
$ comm -12 crossSeq.maternal.sp.gene crossSeq. paternal.sp.
gene > crossSeq.parentShare.gene
$ awk 'NR==FNR{pat[$1]=$0; next} $1 in pat{print pat[$1]}'
crossSeq.maternal.sp.gene.ReadCount crossSeq.parentShare.gene
> crossSeq.parentShare.maternal.sp.gene.ReadCount
$ awk 'NR==FNR{pat[$1]=$0; next} $1 in pat{print pat[$1]}'
crossSeq.paternal.sp.gene.ReadCount crossSeq.parentShare.gene
> crossSeq.parentShare.paternal.sp.gene.ReadCount
$ awk 'NR==FNR{pat[$1]=$3; next} $1 in pat{maternalContr=pat
[$1]/($3+pat[$1]); print $1"\t"maternalContr"\t"1-maternal-
Contr}' crossSeq.parentShare.maternal.sp.gene.ReadCount
crossSeq.parentShare.paternal.sp.gene.ReadCount > crossSeq.
parentShare.contribution
```

2. Calculate the contributions for genes with maternal- or paternal-specific SNPs

```
comm -23 crossSeq.maternal.sp.gene crossSeq. paternal.sp.gene
> crossSeq.maternal.gene
$ awk 'NR==FNR{pat[$1]; next} $1 in pat{if($2>$3){avgREFp=
$2-$3;}else{avgREFp=$2}; maternalContr=$3/($3+avgREFp); print
$0"\t"maternalContr"\t"1-maternalContr;} ' crossSeq.maternal.
```

```
gene crossSeq.maternal.sp.gene.ReadCount > crossSeq.maternal.
contribution
comm -13 crossSeq.maternal.sp.gene crossSeq. paternal.sp.gene
> crossSeq.paternal.gene
$ awk 'NR==FNR{pat[$1]; next} $1 in pat{if($2>$3){avgREFm=
$2-$3;}else{avgREFm=$2}; paternalContr=$3/($3+avgREFm);print
$0"\t"1-paternalContr"\t"paternalContr;} ' crossSeq.paternal.
gene crossSeq.paternal.sp.gene.ReadCount > crossSeq.paternal.
contribution
```

References

1. Wang X, Miller DC, Harman R, Antczak DF, Clark AG (2013) Paternally expressed genes predominate in the placenta. Proc Natl Acad Sci U S A 110:10705–10710

2. Peters J (2014) The role of genomic imprinting in biology and disease: an expanding view. Nat Rev Genet 15:517–530

3. Adams S, Vinkenoog R, Spielman M, Dickinson HG, Scott RJ (2000) Parent-of-origin effects on seed development in Arabidopsis thaliana require DNA methylation. Development 127:2493–2502

4. Autran D, Baroux C, Raissig MT, Lenormand T, Wittig M, Grob S et al (2011) Maternal epigenetic pathways control parental contributions to Arabidopsis early embryogenesis. Cell 145:707–719

5. Tadros W, Lipshitz HD (2009) The maternal-to-zygotic transition: a play in two acts. Development 136:3033–3042

6. Grimanelli D, Perotti E, Ramirez J, Leblanc O (2005) Timing of the maternal-to-zygotic transition during early seed development in maize. Plant Cell 17:1061–1072

7. Pillot M, Baroux C, Vazquez MA, Autran D, Leblanc O, Vielle-Calzada JP et al (2010) Embryo and endosperm inherit distinct chromatin and transcriptional states from the female gametes in Arabidopsis. Plant Cell 22:307–320

8. Del Toro-De Leon G, Garcia-Aguilar M, Gillmor CS (2014) Non-equivalent contributions of maternal and paternal genomes to early plant embryogenesis. Nature 514:624–627

9. Nodine MD, Bartel DP (2012) Maternal and paternal genomes contribute equally to the transcriptome of early plant embryos. Nature 482:94–97

10. Xiang D, Venglat P, Tibiche C, Yang H, Risseeuw E, Cao Y et al (2011) Genome-wide analysis reveals gene expression and metabolic network dynamics during embryo development in Arabidopsis. Plant Physiol 156:346–356

11. Del Fabbro C, Scalabrin S, Morgante M, Giorgi FM (2013) An extensive evaluation of read trimming effects on Illumina NGS data analysis. PLoS One 8:e85024

12. Joshi N, Fass J (2011) Sickle: a sliding-window, adaptive, quality-based trimming tool for FastQ files (Version 1.33) [Software]. https://github.com/najoshi/sickle.

13. Langmead B, Salzberg SL (2012) Fast gapped-read alignment with Bowtie 2. Nat Methods 9:357–359

Chapter 15

Single-Cell Transcriptome Analysis Using SINCERA Pipeline

Minzhe Guo and Yan Xu

Abstract

Genome-scale single-cell biology has recently emerged as a powerful technology with important implications for both basic and medical research. There are urgent needs for the development of computational methods or analytic pipelines to facilitate large amounts of single-cell RNA-Seq data analysis. Here, we present a detailed protocol for SINCERA (*SIN*gle *CE*ll *RNA-Seq* profiling *A*nalysis), a generally applicable analytic pipeline for processing single-cell data from a whole organ or sorted cells. The pipeline supports the analysis for the identification of major cell types, cell type-specific gene signatures, and driving forces of given cell types. In this chapter, we provide step-by-step instructions for the functions and features of SINCERA together with application examples to provide a practical guide for the research community. SINCERA is implemented in R, licensed under the GNU General Public License v3, and freely available from CCHMC PBGE website, https://research.cchmc.org/pbge/sincera.html.

Key words Single-cell, RNA-Seq, Pipeline, Cell type, Signature gene, Driving force

1 Introduction

Single cells are the fundamental units of life. Recent advances in high-throughput cell isolation and sequencing at the single-cell level enable studying individual transcriptomes of large numbers of cells in parallel, providing new insights into the diversity of cell types, rare cells and cell lineage relationships that has been difficult to resolve in genomic data from bulk tissue samples [1–8]. While the single cell research field is still in its early stages, it has already made a strong impact on many fields in biology and led to great improvements in our fundamental understanding of human diseases [9–17]. We believe that the demand of single cell analytic tools will continue to grow in the future as broad applications of single cell transcriptomics in biological and medical researches.

While the future of single-cell next-generation sequencing based genomic/transcriptomic studies is promising, it comes with new and specific analytical challenges including the identification and characterization of unknown cell types, handling the confounding factors such as batch and cell cycle effects, and addressing

Yejun Wang and Ming-an Sun (eds.), *Transcriptome Data Analysis: Methods and Protocols*, Methods in Molecular Biology, vol. 1751, https://doi.org/10.1007/978-1-4939-7710-9_15, © Springer Science+Business Media, LLC 2018

the cellular heterogeneity in complex biological systems, just to name a few [18–22]. Recently, a number of methods specifically designed for single-cell RNA-Seq (scRNA-Seq) analysis have been introduced including BackSPIN [15], SNN-Cliq [23], and RaceID [24] for cell cluster identification; scLVM [22] for confounding factor handling; Seurat [25] for spatial reconstruction of scRNA-Seq data, cell cluster identification, and expression pattern visualization; SAMstrt [26] and SCDE [20] for single-cell differential expression analysis; and Monocle [21], Wanderlust [27], SCUBA [28], Waterfall [29], StemID [16], and SLICE [30] for extracting lineage relationships from scRNA-Seq and modeling the dynamic changes associated with cellular biological processes. Here, we present SINCERA [31], a top-to-bottom single cell analytic tool set designed for the practical usages of the research community. Specifically, the pipeline enables investigators to analyze scRNA-Seq data using standard desktop/laptop computers to conduct data filtering, normalization, clustering, cell type identification, gene signature prediction, transcriptional regulatory network construction, and identification of driving forces (key nodes) for each cell type. We have successfully applied SINCERA to multiple scRNA-Seq datasets from normal developmental lung and various pathological states from both mouse and human, demonstrating SINCERA's general utility and accuracy [31–33].

2   Materials

The entire SINCERA pipeline was implemented in R. The execution requires the following hardware and software.

1. A standard desktop or laptop computer with Windows, Mac OS X, or Linux operating system.

2. R statistical computing environment (version 3.2.0 or later) from The Comprehensive R Archive Network (https://cran.r-project.org/).

3. Install R and Bioconductor packages into the R environment, including Biobase [34], ROCR [35], RobustRankAggreg [36], G1DBN [37], igraph [38], ggplot2 [39], ggdendro (https://cran.r-project.org/web/packages/ggdendro), plyr [40], and zoo [41].

4. Download SINCERA scripts from https://research.cchmc.org/pbge/sincera.html.

3   Methods

SINCERA consists of four major analytic components: preprocessing, cell type identification, gene signature prediction, and driving

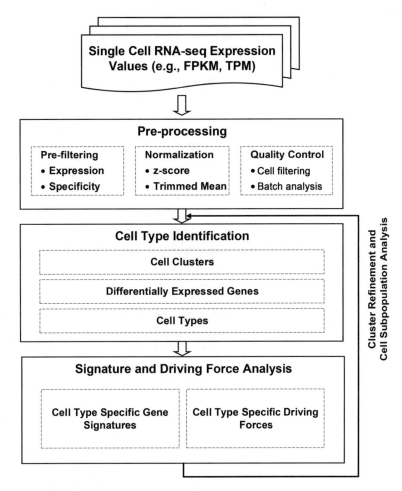

Fig. 1 Schematic flow of the SINCERA protocol (Adapted from Fig. 1 in Guo et al. [31])

force analysis (Fig 1). The pipeline takes RNA-Seq expression values (e.g., FPKM [42] or TPM [43]) from heterogeneous single cell populations as inputs, and it outputs a clustering scheme of cells, differentially expressed genes for each cell cluster, enriched cell type annotations for each cluster, refined cell type-specific gene signature, and cell type-specific rankings of transcription factors. SINCERA is a comprehensive toolset with a variety of options for key analytic steps, many of which can be run independently of one another. To facilitate ease of reference for beginner users, we have marked essential steps with *. In the rest of this chapter, we dissect the functional features of SINCERA into the four components and describe the usages of each component step by step. R functions in SINCERA are depicted in italic font.

3.1 Preprocessing

The preprocessing steps include data transformation and normalization, prefiltering cells with low quality, and prefiltering genes with low expression abundancy and selectivity as described below.

1. *The analysis starts with running the *construct* function to create an R S4 object, which will hold all the data and analysis results. The function takes two parameters as inputs: "exprfile" and "samplefile". The "exprfile" specifies the full path to a gene expression profile matrix where rows are genes and columns are individual cells (*see* **Note 1**). The "samplefile" parameter specifies the full path to a table that contains a single column describing the sample information (e.g., biological replicates or batch difference) of individual cells. Figure 2 shows the required formats of the two input files.

2. The CCHMC single cell core inspects each individual cell under microscope after capture and prior to lysis. This quality control (QC) step is important in filtering out libraries made from empty wells or wells with excess debris. In addition, we run the *filterLowQualityCells* function of SINCERA to further identify and remove low quality cells. The key parameters of running this function include: "min.expression", which specifies the minimum expression value for a gene to be considered an expressed gene, and "min.genes", which specifies the lower bound of the number of expressed genes in a cell. This function identifies and removes cells with few expressed genes. The default value for the "min.expression" parameter is 1 FPKM/ TPM and for the "min.genes" parameter is 500.

3. Use *filterContaminatedCells* function to remove potential contaminated cells based on the coexpression of known marker genes of two distinct cell types, such as the coexpression of mouse lung epithelial marker *Epcam* and mouse lung endothelial cell marker *Pecam1*. Users can specify the marker genes of the first cell type and of the second cell type in the "markers.1" and "markers.2" parameter, respectively. This step can repeat multiple times. For each cell type, we suggest using only highly specific markers for contamination detection.

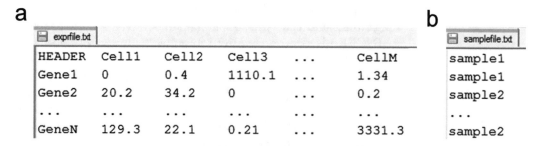

a

exprfile.txt					
HEADER	Cell1	Cell2	Cell3	...	CellM
Gene1	0	0.4	1110.1	...	1.34
Gene2	20.2	34.2	0	...	0.2
...	...	...	...	...	...
GeneN	129.3	22.1	0.21	...	3331.3

b

samplefile.txt
sample1
sample1
sample2
...
sample2

Fig. 2 Formats of the input files to the SINCERA pipeline. (**a**) Format of expression profile table. (**b**) Format of sample description table. The number of rows in the sample description table is the same as the number of cells in the expression profile table. Both files are tab delimited text files

4. *Use *prefilterGenes* function to filter out non- or low-expressed genes, as well as genes that are expressed in less than a certain number of cells per sample preparation. By default, genes expressed (>5 FPKM/TPM) in less than two cells will be filtered out by this function.

5. *Use *expr.minimum* function to set a minimum expression value. As part of the preprocessing step, we transformed FPKM/TPM values less than or equal to 0.01–0.01 in order to eliminate "zero"s from the follow up data transformation and analysis. The default minimum value is 0.01 FPKM/TPM.

6. Run *batch.analysis* function to identify batch differences. This function plots the quantiles of gene expression in individual cells from different batches, and compares the distribution of gene expression among batches using MA plot, Q–Q plot, and cell correlation and distance measure [31].

7. *Normalization methods are applied to reduce batch effect and enable expression level comparisons within or across sample preparations. SINCERA provides both gene level and cell level normalizations. For gene level normalization, *normalization.zscore* function is applied to each gene expression profile for per-sample z-score transformation (*see* **Note 2**). For cell level normalizations, we use the trimmed mean. If starting with normalized expression data (e.g., FPKM or TPM), cell level normalization is not always necessary.

8. *Run *cluster.geneSelection* function to select genes with a certain level of expression specificity for cell type identification. This specificity filter [31] removes genes unselectively expressed across all cell types (e.g., housekeeping genes) and keeps genes with a certain degree of cell type selective expression. The default specificity threshold is set as 0.7. The main purpose of this step is to select expression profiles that are potentially informative about cell types/states and remove genes that may increase noise in the cell type identification step (*see* **Note 3**).

3.2 Cell Type Identification

Cell clustering and cell type identification is a key step in the pipeline and directly influences all downstream analysis. SINCERA starts with an unsupervised hierarchical clustering of the cells using the selected expression profiles. Use of an unsupervised hierarchical clustering approach does not impose prerequisite external biological knowledge, nor does it require preset knowledge of the number of clusters; therefore, it is capable of discovering novel cell types. Multiple iterations using more than one clustering methods are usually required for cell cluster refinement (*see* **Note 4**).

1. *Run *cluster.assignment* function to assign cells to initial clusters. The default algorithm uses hierarchical clustering with average linkage, Pearson's correlation based distance

measurement, and z-score transformed expression values of the selected genes.

2. *Run *plotMarkers* function to check the quality of the obtained clustering scheme and inspect the expression patterns of a number of known markers across cell clusters. A scattered and/or overlapping expression pattern of cell type marker genes across different cell clusters may suggest a low quality clustering scheme. In this case, we recommend using *cluster.assignment* function with a different parameter setting to redefine cell clusters. This process may need to be iterated several times to achieve better separation.

3. Run the *cluster.permutation.analysis* function to perform a cluster membership permutation analysis [31] to determine cluster significance. SINCERA implements several quality control or internal validation steps; this is one of them, used to check quality of clustering schemes.

4. *Once cell clusters have been defined, use *cluster.diffgenes* function to identify differentially expressed genes in each cluster. For each cell cluster, this function uses one-tailed Welch's t test or Wilcoxon test to compare the gene expression in a given cell cluster to the corresponding gene expression in all other cells, and genes with p-value less than a threshold are identified as differentially expressed genes for the cluster. One can also choose binomial or negative-binomial probability test in this step. The default threshold is 0.05.

5. Next, run *celltype.enrichment* function to predict cell type for each cluster (*see* **Note 5**). SINCERA has built a precompiled cell type and gene association table using experimental expression data obtained from EBI expression atlas (https://www.ebi.ac.uk/gxa). Cell type prediction is based on the enrichment of cell type annotations significantly associated with differentially expressed genes of the given cluster using a one-tailed Fisher's exact test.

6. Once cell clusters have been defined, use *plotMarkers* function to visualize the expression patterns of known cell type markers in order to cross validate the predicted cell type, i.e., to check whether they are selectively expressed in their defined cell clusters.

7. Run *celltype.validation* function to perform a rank-aggregation-based quantitative assessment of the consistency between mapped cell type and the expression pattern of known cell type marker genes. Figure 3 demonstrates the application of SINCERA to identify major cell types at E16.5 mouse lung and to validate the cell type assignment using known markers.

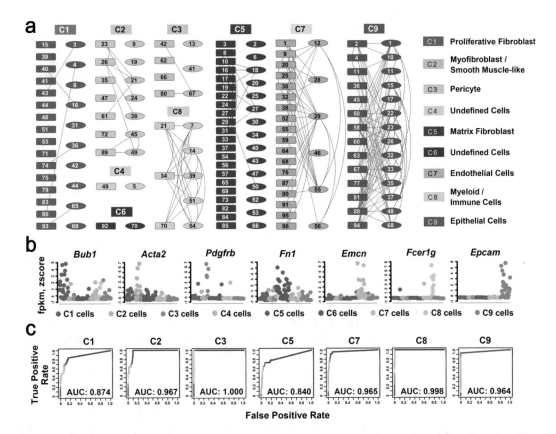

Fig. 3 Identification and validation of major lung cell types at E16.5 mouse lung (Adapted from Figs. 2 and 3 in Guo et al. [31]). (**a**) Cells ($n = 148$) from two sample preparations from fetal mouse lung at E16.5 [31] were assigned into nine clusters via hierarchical clustering using average linkage and centered Pearson's correlation. Each color represents a distinct cell cluster, labeled as C1–C9. The rectangles represent single lung cells from the first preparation and the ellipses consist of single cells from a second independent preparation. Connection lines indicate the z-score correlation between the two cells ≥ 0.05. The blue lines connect cells within the same preparation, while the red lines connect cells across preparations. (**b**) Expression patterns of representative known cell type markers were used to validate the correct assignment of major lung cell types at E16.5. Expression levels were normalized by per-sample z-score transformation. (**c**) Receiver Operating Characteristic curves of the rank-aggregation-based validation showed a high consistency between the cell type assignments and the expression patterns of known cell type-specific markers

3.3 Cell Type-Specific Signature Gene Analysis

We define cell type-specific gene signature as a group of genes uniquely or selectively expressed in a given cell type. Once cell types have been defined, the analysis proceeds with the identification of cell type-specific gene signatures using the following functions.

1. Collect positive and negative marker genes for each mapped cell type. Use *setCellTypeMarkers* function to add the collected markers into SINCERA.

2. *Run the *signature.prediction* function to predict cell type signature genes. The basic level of prediction defines

differentially expressed genes of the given cell type as the signature genes. For more advanced prediction, the *signature. prediction* function uses four features [31] to define cell type-specific signature genes, including common gene metric (genes shared by the cluster cells), unique gene metric (genes selectively expressed in the cluster cells), test statistic metric (group mean comparison between cluster cells and all the other cells), and synthetic profile similarity (genes correlating with the model profile of the given cluster). When the marker genes of a cell type are available, the *signature.prediction* function uses a logistic regression model to integrate the four metrics for ranking prediction of cell-specific signatures [31]. Nevertheless, marker genes may not be always available, especially for novel cell types. In such cases, the *signature.prediction* function predicts signature by using additional filters to refine differentially expressed genes, including a frequency filter and a fold change filter. The frequency filter selects genes expressed in at least a certain percentage of the cells within the defined cluster. The fold change filter selects genes with a certain degree of average expression enrichment in the given cluster compared to the cluster with its second highest average expression. The default frequency and fold change threshold is 30% and 1.5, respectively.

3. Use *plotHeatmap* function to visualize the expression of the predicted signature genes across cell types (clusters). This allows a visual inspection of the selective expression of the predicted signature genes in the defined cell types.

4. Run *signature.validation* function to validate the signature prediction using a repeated random subsampling approach [31]. Essentially, this approach validates the predicted signature by assessing its classification accuracy in distinguishing the cells of the given cell type from cells of other types.

3.4 Cell Type-Specific Key Regulator Prediction

Identification of the key regulators controlling cell fate is essential for understanding complex biological systems. SINCERA utilizes a transcriptional regulatory network (TRN) approach to establish the relationships between transcription factors (TFs) and target genes (TGs) based on their expression-based regulatory potential and identify the key TFs for a given cell type by measuring the importance of each node in the constructed TRN.

1. Run *drivingfoce.selectTFs* function to select candidate transcription factors for the prediction. The function selects the union of cell type-specific differentially expressed TFs (e.g., p-value of one-tailed Welch's t test <0.05) and commonly expressed TFs (e.g., expressed in at least 80% of the cell type) as candidates. Note that here we do not require a key regulator for a given cell type to be differentially expressed in the cell type.

a

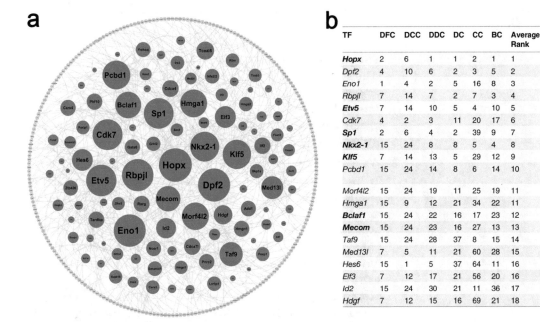

b

TF	DFC	DCC	DDC	DC	CC	BC	Average Rank
Hopx	2	6	1	1	2	1	1
Dpf2	4	10	6	2	3	5	2
Eno1	1	4	2	5	16	8	3
Rbpjl	7	14	7	2	7	3	4
Etv5	7	14	10	5	4	10	5
Cdk7	4	2	3	11	20	17	6
Sp1	2	6	4	2	39	9	7
Nkx2-1	15	24	8	8	5	4	8
Klf5	7	14	13	5	29	12	9
Pcbd1	15	24	14	8	6	14	10
Morf4l2	15	24	19	11	25	19	11
Hmga1	15	9	12	21	34	22	11
Bclaf1	15	24	22	16	17	23	12
Mecom	15	24	23	16	27	13	13
Taf9	15	24	28	37	8	15	14
Med13l	7	5	11	21	60	28	15
Hes6	15	1	5	37	64	11	16
Elf3	7	12	17	21	56	20	16
Id2	15	24	30	21	11	36	17
Hdgf	7	12	15	16	69	21	18

Fig. 4 Prediction of E16.5 mouse lung epithelial specific driving force (Adapted from Fig. 6 and Table 1 in Guo et al. [31]). (**a**) Rank importance of transcription factors (TFs) in the largest connected component (LCC) of epithelial specific transcriptional regulatory network (TRN). The sizes of the TF nodes are proportional to their average-ranked node importance. The LCC of epithelial TRN is comprised of 348 nodes and 432 edges. The nodes in red are TFs and the nodes in grey are differentially expressed genes in epithelial cells and are not TFs. The edges were established using the first-order conditional dependence approach described in the Guo et al. [31] with a cutoff at 0.05. (**b**) Top 20 predicted key TFs for lung epithelial cells at E16.5 based on the integration of six TF importance metrics. *DC* ranking based on degree centrality, *CC* ranking based on closeness centrality, *BC* ranking based on betweenness centrality, *DFC* ranking based on disruptive fragmentation centrality, *DCC* ranking based on disruptive connection centrality, *DDC* ranking based on disruptive distance centrality. All ranks are in decreasing order of the TF importance values. TFs in bold font are associated with lung-related mouse phenotypes. TRN is plotted using cytoscape 2.8 (http:/www.cytoscape.org/)

2. Use *drivingforce.selectTGs* function to select cell type-specific differentially expressed genes or signature genes as candidate target genes (TGs).

3. Use *drivingforce.inferTRN* function to infer a TRN using the cell type-specific expression patterns of the selected candidate TFs and TGs. The "edge.threshold" parameter is used to select significant TF-TF or TF-TG interactions (*see* **Note 6**) for building the network. The default threshold is set to 0.05 (*see* **Note 7**).

4. Use *drivingforce.rankTFs* function to rank TFs based on their importance to the inferred TRN (*see* **Note 8**). Top ranked TFs are predicted as key regulators (driving force) for the given cell type. Figure 4 demonstrates of using SINCERA to predict key TFs in E16.5 mouse lung epithelial cells.

4   Notes

1. The pipeline takes aligned and quantified RNA-Seq expression values (e.g., FPKM or TPM) as inputs. Functions related to sequencing data mapping, alignment, quantification, and annotation are not part of the pipeline, and they can be processed using widely available software such as Tophat [44, 45], BWA [46], Cufflinks [42], and RSEM [43].

2. We noticed that, typically, in a scRNA-Seq dataset, individual genes can have different levels of baseline expression, which means that a cell type selective marker may have nonzero expression in cells other than its defined cell type, but its expression amplitude is usually much higher in the selective cell type than in other cell types. The *normalization.zscore* function scales the expression of individual genes using a *z*-score transformation in order to better reveal their major expression patterns and suppress the unnecessary variations associated with the scRNA-Seq data. Performing within-sample *z*-score transformation is based on the assumption that cell type distribution is roughly the same among replicates. If this assumption cannot be guaranteed (e.g., there is a large batch difference among different replicates), a global *z*-score transformation should be used. Of note, the *z*-score transformed expression values are mainly used in the cell type identification step and the visualization of gene expression patterns, but not in differential expression analysis.

3. The *cluster.geneSelection* function also provides other criteria for informative gene selection, including coefficient of variance and average expression across all cells, which have been utilized in existing scRNA-Seq analyses [12, 22]. The *specificity.thresholdSelection* function in SINCERA can be used to determine the specificity threshold. This function measures the per-sample specificity of a set of ribosomal genes based on Ribosome pathway annotation (KEGG PATHWAY: hsa03010), and then chooses a criterion that can filter out at least 95% of the ribosomal genes.

4. We compared multiple clustering algorithms using a variety of independent scRNA-Seq datasets [31] and showed that hierarchical clustering, while may not always be the best way, is generally applicable and easy to use. Therefore, hierarchical clustering is suitable for biologists to use as one of the tools for initial cell clustering identification [31]. In addition to the default clustering method, we also include hierarchical clustering with ward linkage [47], consensus clustering [48, 49], and tight clustering [50] as optional cluster determination methods in the pipeline. Users can choose different clustering methods

for cell cluster identification by setting the "clustering. method" parameter in the *cluster.assignment* function. For advanced users, comparing different methods and adjusting parameters to achieve optimized results are encouraged.

5. The cell cluster identification and cell type assignment are the bottlenecks in current scRNA-Seq analysis. It requires us to extract cell type relevant information from multiple sources, including the expression patterns of known marker genes and functional annotations enriched by the cluster specific differentially expressed genes. Knowledge integration by an expert is usually required to determine the cell type of a given cell cluster at the end. To our knowledge, there are multiple tools for gene sets enrichment analysis, e.g., DAVID [51] and ToppGene [52], but lack of tools for cell type enrichment analysis. To facilitate the general usage of the pipeline, we implemented *celltype.enrichment* function in SINCERA as an attempt to automate the cell type prediction. The current version of cell type annotations is based on the open source gene expression data from EBI Expression Atlas (https://www.ebi.ac.uk/gxa); bias and incompleteness from the collection of individual experimental sources are inevitable. We recommend the use of it for initial cell type screening, together with functional enrichment analysis using cluster specific differentially expressed genes, and curation and knowledge integration by experts to refine the cell type mapping. We foresee that single cell transcriptome analyses will largely improve cell type prediction by providing a high resolution and unbiased cell type separation and associated signature identification for lung and other organs.

6. For the transcriptional regulatory network (TRN) construction, we focus on identifying the relationships between TF-TF (transcription factor and its partners/cofactors) and TF-TG (transcription factor and its target genes). The possible feedback regulations from target genes to TFs and TF autoregulations are not considered in the present implementation of SINCERA. Regulatory relationships are established based on first-order conditional dependence of gene expression [31], adapted from the inference of first-order conditional dependence Directed Acyclic Graph (DAG) in [37].

7. The inferred TRN may consist of multiple connected components. The largest connected component (LCC) is the one that has the largest number of nodes among all connected components. If the LCC of the inferred TRN is not large enough, which means that the number of nodes in LCC is less than a certain percentage (e.g., 80%) of the total number of selected TFs and TGs for TRN inference, this indicates that the number of interactions is insufficient to build the TRN. The

drivingforce.inferTRN function needs to be reexecuted with a higher threshold to build the TRN using more interactions. The *drivingforce.getLCC* function can be used to assess whether a large enough LCC exists in the inferred TRN.

8. To identify cell type-specific driving force, we measure and rank the importance of TFs in the cell type-specific TRN based on the integration of six TF importance metrics, including degree centrality, closeness centrality, betweenness centrality, disruptive fragmentation centrality, disruptive connection centrality, and disruptive distance centrality. Details about the six metrics can be found in Guo et al. [31]. Individual metrics provide local views of the importance of a node to the network, and their integration can provide a better global view of the node importance in the network. In the current setting, only the TFs in the LCC of the inferred TRN are included in the TF ranking, and only the LCC is used to calculate the values of the six metrics for each TF.

Acknowledgment

This work was supported by the National Heart, Lung, and Blood Institute of National Institutes of Health (http://www.nhlbi.nih.gov, grants U01HL122642 (LungMAP), U01 HL110967 (LRRC), and R01 HL105433). The funders had no role in study design, data collection and analysis, decision to publish, or preparation of the manuscript.

References

1. Tang F, Barbacioru C, Wang Y, Nordman E, Lee C, Xu N, Wang X, Bodeau J, Tuch BB, Siddiqui A et al (2009) mRNA-Seq whole-transcriptome analysis of a single cell. Nat Methods 6:377–382

2. Tang F, Barbacioru C, Bao S, Lee C, Nordman E, Wang X, Lao K, Surani MA (2010) Tracing the derivation of embryonic stem cells from the inner cell mass by single-cell RNA-Seq analysis. Cell Stem Cell 6:468–478

3. Qiu S, Luo S, Evgrafov O, Li R, Schroth GP, Levitt P, Knowles JA, Wang K (2012) Single-neuron RNA-Seq: technical feasibility and reproducibility. Front Genet 3:124

4. Ramskold D, Luo S, Wang YC, Li R, Deng Q, Faridani OR, Daniels GA, Khrebtukova I, Loring JF, Laurent LC et al (2012) Full-length mRNA-Seq from single-cell levels of RNA and individual circulating tumor cells. Nat Biotechnol 30:777–782

5. Islam S, Kjallquist U, Moliner A, Zajac P, Fan JB, Lonnerberg P, Linnarsson S (2011) Characterization of the single-cell transcriptional landscape by highly multiplex RNA-Seq. Genome Res 21:1160–1167

6. Narsinh KH, Sun N, Sanchez-Freire V, Lee AS, Almeida P, Hu S, Jan T, Wilson KD, Leong D, Rosenberg J et al (2011) Single cell transcriptional profiling reveals heterogeneity of human induced pluripotent stem cells. J Clin Invest 121:1217–1221

7. Shalek AK, Satija R, Adiconis X, Gertner RS, Gaublomme JT, Raychowdhury R, Schwartz S, Yosef N, Malboeuf C, Lu D et al (2013) Single-cell transcriptomics reveals bimodality in expression and splicing in immune cells. Nature 498:236–240

8. Wills QF, Livak KJ, Tipping AJ, Enver T, Goldson AJ, Sexton DW, Holmes C (2013) Single-cell gene expression analysis reveals genetic

associations masked in whole-tissue experiments. Nat Biotechnol 31:748–752

9. Wang Y, Waters J, Leung ML, Unruh A, Roh W, Shi X, Chen K, Scheet P, Vattathil S, Liang H et al (2014) Clonal evolution in breast cancer revealed by single nucleus genome sequencing. Nature 512:155–160

10. Hanchate NK, Kondoh K, Lu Z, Kuang D, Ye X, Qiu X, Pachter L, Trapnell C, Buck LB (2015) Single-cell transcriptomics reveals receptor transformations during olfactory neurogenesis. Science 350:1251–1255

11. Lee JH, Daugharthy ER, Scheiman J, Kalhor R, Ferrante TC, Terry R, Turczyk BM, Yang JL, Lee HS, Aach J et al (2015) Fluorescent in situ sequencing (FISSEQ) of RNA for gene expression profiling in intact cells and tissues. Nat Protoc 10:442–458

12. Macosko EZ, Basu A, Satija R, Nemesh J, Shekhar K, Goldman M, Tirosh I, Bialas AR, Kamitaki N, Martersteck EM et al (2015) Highly parallel genome-wide expression profiling of individual cells using nanoliter droplets. Cell 161:1202–1214

13. Saadatpour A, Lai S, Guo G, Yuan GC (2015) Single-cell analysis in cancer genomics. Trends Genet 31:576–586

14. Vaughan AE, Brumwell AN, Xi Y, Gotts JE, Brownfield DG, Treutlein B, Tan K, Tan V, Liu FC, Looney MR et al (2015) Lineage-negative progenitors mobilize to regenerate lung epithelium after major injury. Nature 517:621–625

15. Zeisel A, Munoz-Manchado AB, Codeluppi S, Lonnerberg P, La Manno G, Jureus A, Marques S, Munguba H, He L, Betsholtz C et al (2015) Brain structure. Cell types in the mouse cortex and hippocampus revealed by single-cell RNA-Seq. Science 347:1138–1142

16. Grün D, Muraro MJ, Boisset JC, Wiebrands K, Lyubimova A, Dharmadhikari G, van den Born M, van Es J, Jansen E, Clevers H et al (2016) De novo prediction of stem cell identity using single-cell transcriptome data. Cell Stem Cell 19:266–277

17. Shekhar K, Lapan SW, Whitney IE, Tran NM, Macosko EZ, Kowalczyk M, Adiconis X, Levin JZ, Nemesh J, Goldman M et al (2016) Comprehensive classification of retinal bipolar neurons by single-cell transcriptomics. Cell 166 (1308–1323):e1330

18. Kim JK, Marioni JC (2013) Inferring the kinetics of stochastic gene expression from single-cell RNA-sequencing data. Genome Biol 14: R7

19. Brennecke P, Anders S, Kim JK, Kolodziejczyk AA, Zhang X, Proserpio V, Baying B, Benes V, Teichmann SA, Marioni JC et al (2013) Accounting for technical noise in single-cell RNA-Seq experiments. Nat Methods 10:1093–1095

20. Kharchenko PV, Silberstein L, Scadden DT (2014) Bayesian approach to single-cell differential expression analysis. Nat Methods 11:740–742

21. Trapnell C, Cacchiarelli D, Grimsby J, Pokharel P, Li S, Morse M, Lennon NJ, Livak KJ, Mikkelsen TS, Rinn JL (2014) The dynamics and regulators of cell fate decisions are revealed by pseudotemporal ordering of single cells. Nat Biotechnol 32:381–386

22. Buettner F, Natarajan KN, Casale FP, Proserpio V, Scialdone A, Theis FJ, Teichmann SA, Marioni JC, Stegle O (2015) Computational analysis of cell-to-cell heterogeneity in single-cell RNA-Sequencing data reveals hidden subpopulations of cells. Nat Biotechnol 33:155–160

23. Xu C, Su Z (2015) Identification of cell types from single-cell transcriptomes using a novel clustering method. Bioinformatics 31:1974–1980

24. Grun D, Lyubimova A, Kester L, Wiebrands K, Basak O, Sasaki N, Clevers H, van Oudenaarden A (2015) Single-cell messenger RNA sequencing reveals rare intestinal cell types. Nature 525:251–255

25. Satija R, Farrell JA, Gennert D, Schier AF, Regev A (2015) Spatial reconstruction of single-cell gene expression data. Nat Biotechnol 33:495–502

26. Katayama S, Tohonen V, Linnarsson S, Kere J (2013) SAMstrt: statistical test for differential expression in single-cell transcriptome with spike-in normalization. Bioinformatics 29:2943–2945

27. Bendall SC, Davis KL, Amirel AD, Tadmor MD, Simonds EF, Chen TJ, Shenfeld DK, Nolan GP, Pe'er D (2014) Single-cell trajectory detection uncovers progression and regulatory coordination in human B cell development. Cell 157:714–725

28. Marco E, Karp RL, Guo G, Robson P, Hart AH, Trippa L, Yuan GC (2014) Bifurcation analysis of single-cell gene expression data reveals epigenetic landscape. Proc Natl Acad Sci U S A 111:E5643–E5650

29. Shin J, Berg DA, Zhu YH, Shin JY, Song J, Bonaguidi MA, Enikolopov G, Nauen DW, Christian KM, Ming GL et al (2015) Single-cell RNA-seq with waterfall reveals molecular cascades underlying adult neurogenesis. Cell Stem Cell 17:360–372

30. Guo M, Bao EL, Wagner M, Whitsett JA, Xu Y (2017) SLICE: determining cell differentiation and lineage based on single cell entropy. Nucleic Acids Res 45(7):e54

31. Guo M, Wang H, Potter SS, Whitsett JA, Xu Y (2015) SINCERA: a pipeline for single-cell RNA-seq profiling analysis. PLoS Comput Biol 11:e1004575

32. Du Y, Guo M, Whitsett JA, Xu Y (2015) 'LungGENS': a web-based tool for mapping single-cell gene expression in the developing lung. Thorax 70:1092–1094

33. Xu Y, Mizuno T, Sridharan A, Du Y, Guo M, Tang J, Wikenheiser-Brokamp KA, Perl A-KT, Funari VA, Gokey JJ et al (2016) Single-cell RNA sequencing identifies diverse roles of epithelial cells in idiopathic pulmonary fibrosis. JCI Insight 1:e90558

34. Huber W, Carey VJ, Gentleman R, Anders S, Carlson M, Carvalho BS, Bravo HC, Davis S, Gatto L, Girke T et al (2015) Orchestrating high-throughput genomic analysis with bioconductor. Nat Methods 12:115–121

35. Sing T, Sander O, Beerenwinkel N, Lengauer T (2005) ROCR: visualizing classifier performance in R. Bioinformatics 21:3940–3941

36. Kolde R, Laur S, Adler P, Vilo J (2012) Robust rank aggregation for gene list integration and meta-analysis. Bioinformatics 28:573–580

37. Lebre S (2009) Inferring dynamic genetic networks with low order independencies. Stat Appl Genet Mol Biol 8:Article 9

38. Csardi G, Nepusz T (2006) The igraph software package for complex network research. InterJ Comp Syst 1695:1–9

39. Wickham H (2009) ggplot2: elegant graphics for data analysis. Springer, New York, NY

40. Wickham H (2011) The split-apply-combine strategy for data analysis. J Stat Softw 40:1–29

41. Zeileis A, Grothendieck G (2005) zoo: S3 infrastructure for regular and irregular time series. J Stat Softw 14. https://doi.org/10.18637/jss.v014.i06

42. Trapnell C, Williams BA, Pertea G, Mortazavi A, Kwan G, van Baren MJ, Salzberg SL, Wold BJ, Pachter L (2010) Transcript assembly and quantification by RNA-Seq reveals unannotated transcripts and isoform switching during cell differentiation. Nat Biotechnol 28:511–515

43. Li B, Dewey CN (2011) RSEM: accurate transcript quantification from RNA-Seq data with or without a reference genome. BMC Bioinformatics 12:323

44. Kim D, Pertea G, Trapnell C, Pimentel H, Kelley R, Salzberg SL (2013) TopHat2: accurate alignment of transcriptomes in the presence of insertions, deletions and gene fusions. Genome Biol 14:R36

45. Trapnell C, Pachter L, Salzberg SL (2009) TopHat: discovering splice junctions with RNA-Seq. Bioinformatics 25:1105–1111

46. Li H, Durbin R (2009) Fast and accurate short read alignment with Burrows-Wheeler transform. Bioinformatics 25:1754–1760

47. Ward JH Jr (1963) Hierarchical grouping to optimize an objective function. J Am Stat Assoc 58:236–244

48. Monti S, Tamayo P, Mesirov JP, Golub TR (2003) Consensus clustering: a resampling-based method for class discovery and visualization of gene expression microarray data. Mach Learn 52:91–118

49. Wilkerson MD, Hayes DN (2010) ConsensusClusterPlus: a class discovery tool with confidence assessments and item tracking. Bioinformatics 26:1572–1573

50. Tseng GC, Wong WH (2005) Tight clustering: a resampling-based approach for identifying stable and tight patterns in data. Biometrics 61:10–16

51. Huang DW, Sherman BT, Lempicki RA (2009) Systematic and integrative analysis of large gene lists using DAVID bioinformatics resources. Nat Protoc 4:44–57

52. Chen J, Bardes EE, Aronow BJ, Jegga AG (2009) ToppGene suite for gene list enrichment analysis and candidate gene prioritization. Nucleic Acids Res 37:W305–W311

Chapter 16

Mathematical Modeling and Deconvolution of Molecular Heterogeneity Identifies Novel Subpopulations in Complex Tissues

Niya Wang, Lulu Chen, and Yue Wang

Abstract

Tissue heterogeneity is both a major confounding factor and an underexploited information source. While a handful of reports have demonstrated the potential of supervised methods to deconvolve tissue heterogeneity, these approaches require a priori information on the marker genes or composition of known subpopulations. To address the critical problem of the absence of validated marker genes for many (including novel) subpopulations, we develop a novel unsupervised deconvolution method, Convex Analysis of Mixtures (CAM), within a well-grounded mathematical framework, to dissect mixed gene expressions in heterogeneous tissue samples. To facilitate the utility of this method, we implement an R-Java CAM package that provides comprehensive analytic functions and graphic user interface (GUI).

Key words Convex analysis of mixture, Data deconvolution, Tissue heterogeneity, Marker genes, Blind source separation

1 Introduction

Tissue heterogeneity, arising from multiple subpopulations within a sample, is both a major confounding factor in studying individual subpopulations and an underexploited information source for characterizing complex tissues [1, 2]. Because the interactions among subpopulations are fundamental to both normal development and disease progression, molecular analysis of subpopulations in their native microenvironment provides the most biologically relevant picture of the in vivo state [3, 4]. Complex tissues can be characterized by the identity, composition, and expression profile of possibly unknown subpopulations [5], where subpopulations are often defined by marker genes (genes whose expressions are exclusively enriched in a particular subpopulation [6, 7], Fig. 1a). Current global profiling methods can neither identify differentially expressed genes among different subpopulations, nor distinguish among the contributions of different subpopulations to a globally measured

Yejun Wang and Ming-an Sun (eds.), *Transcriptome Data Analysis: Methods and Protocols*, Methods in Molecular Biology, vol. 1751, https://doi.org/10.1007/978-1-4939-7710-9_16, © Springer Science+Business Media, LLC 2018

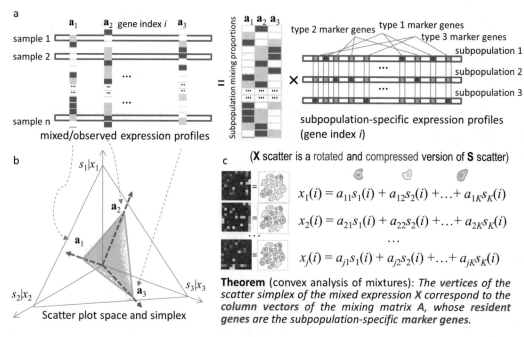

Fig. 1 CAM principles for unsupervised identification of novel subpopulation-specific marker genes

gene expression profile [1, 5]. Thus, it is generally impossible to tell whether expression change reflects a change in subpopulation composition, a change in subpopulation-specific expression, or both.

An experimental solution to mitigate tissue heterogeneity is to isolate subpopulations before molecular profiling by supervised cell sorting or tissue microdissection [1, 8]. However, these methods are biased, costly, inapplicable to previously assayed samples, and may alter the expression values [5, 6]. While some reports have demonstrated the potential of computational methods to resolve tissue heterogeneity, a priori information on the composition [2, 5, 9] or signatures [6, 10–12] of the subpopulations believed to be present is almost exclusively required. Acquiring these prior information relies on experimental solutions and key limitations remain unsolved. Such supervised methods consequently have difficulty detecting subpopulations that are subtle, condition-specific (molecular signatures and cell function are changed but not cell appearance), or previously unknown [3, 13].

To address the critical problem of the absence of validated marker genes for many (including novel) subpopulations, we developed a fully unsupervised computational method (convex analysis of mixtures—CAM) that can identify subpopulation-specific marker genes directly from the original mixed expressions—a nontrivial task. CAM requires no prior information on the number, identity, or composition of the subpopulations present in mixed samples [12], and does not require the presence of pure subpopulations in sample space [14, 15]. Fundamental to the success of our approach is the newly proven mathematical theorems, showing that the scatter simplex of mixed expressions is a rotated and compressed version of the scatter simplex of pure expressions, where the marker genes are located at each vertex (Fig. 1b). CAM works by geometrically identifying the vertices (and their resident genes) of the scatter simplex of globally measured expressions (**Note 1**).

Tissue samples to be analyzed by CAM contain unknown numbers and varying proportions of molecularly distinct subpopulations. Expression of a given gene in a specific subpopulation is modeled as being linearly proportional to the abundance of that subpopulation [5, 6] (without log transformation [16], Fig. 1c). Because many genes can be coexpressed across different subpopulations, CAM instead identifies the subpopulation-specific marker genes by detecting the simplex vertices of mixed expression data (**Note 2**). The minimum description length (MDL) criterion determines the number of subpopulations present [17] (**Note 3**).

2 Materials

To facilitate various applications of CAM method, we developed an R-Java CAM package that provides comprehensive analytic functions and graphic user interface (GUI) to help users readily apply CAM method to their own datasets. The core functions of CAM are implemented in R, while the GUI is in Java, so some prerequisites need to be fulfilled before running the software package.

1. CAM has been tested under Windows, Mac OS X, and Linux operating system, so any of the operating systems is applicable.

2. The latest version of CAM is implemented in Java SE 6 Update 31 and R 2.15.3. The compatible versions of Java and R environments need to be installed.

3. "Runiversal" and "R.matlab" packages need to be installed in the R environment. Runiversal package is used for the communication between R and Java, and R.matlab package is used to read MAT files.

4. Download CAM software from http://mloss.org/software/view/437. Users can simply use GUI to run the software, or run the core R module alone under R environment.

3 Methods

The steps of applying CAM to data analysis are illustrated in the following flowchart (Fig. 2). Users who are interested in the details about the algorithm can find all information in **Note 4**.

3.1 Software

CAM package consists of R and Java modules. The R module is a collection of main and helper functions, each represented by an R

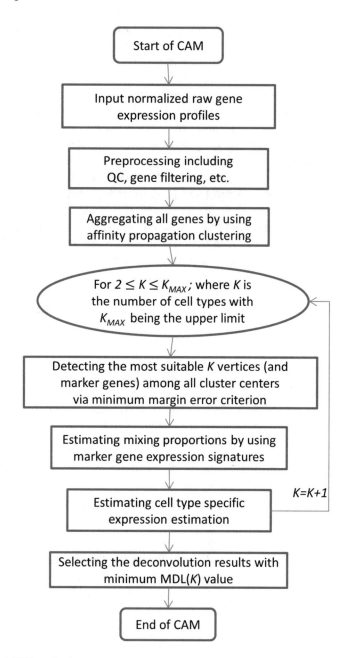

Fig. 2 Flowchart of CAM method

function object and achieving an independent and specific task (Fig. 3). The R module mainly performs various analytic tasks required by CAM: figure plotting, update, or error message generation. The Java module is developed to provide a GUI (Fig. 4).

The R module performs the CAM algorithm and facilitates subsequent analyses including compartment modeling (CM) [18, 19], nonnegative independent component analysis

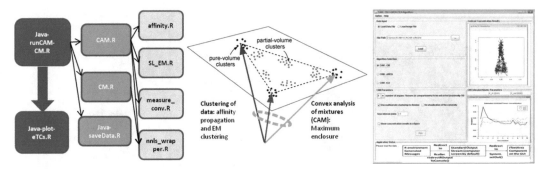

Fig. 3 Schematic and illustrative flowchart of R-Java CAM package

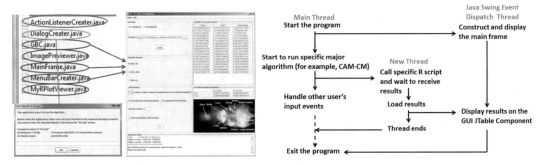

Fig. 4 Interactive Java GUI supported by a multithread design strategy

(nICA) [20], and nonnegative well-grounded component analysis (nWCA) [21, 22]. These tasks are performed by the three main functions: CAM-CM.R, CAM-nICA.R, and CAM-nWCA.R, which can be activated by the three R scripts, namely, Java-run-CAM-CM.R, Java-runCAM-ICA.R, and Java-runCAM-nWCA.R.

After launching the jar file "CAM-Java.jar" by double-clicking it or running the command line "java -jar CAM-Java.jar" in the terminal, a dialogue window will pop up allowing the user to enter the file path of the binary executable file "Rscript.exe", which can be easily found in the installation folder of R. After entering the correct file path, we can see the main frame of the software as Fig. 4.

Here we use a sample dataset—the real DCE-MRI dataset in the software package to show how to use the software to analyze heterogeneous data (**Note 4–6**).

(a) Select "Load Data File" on the main frame and click "…" button.

(b) In the file selection dialog, first select "R / Matlab Data (*.rda, *.mat)" in "Files of Type:", then select one dataset from the following file path "data / data_DCE_MRI/ typical_case. rda". Click "Open" and then click "Load".

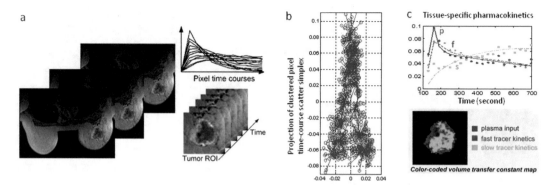

Fig. 5 Application of R-Java CAM to deconvolving dynamic medical image sequence

(c) On the main frame of the software, Select "CAM-CM", set "number of organs" to 3 and time interval to 0.5 min, check the boxes "Use multivariate clustering to denoise", "Do visualization of the convexity", and "Show concentration" results in a figure, and then click "Run".

After about 2–3 min, the results will be shown in the table areas (Fig. 4), together with two figures (Fig. 5b, c) displayed in separated windows.

In this case, the number of compartments 3 is decided by minimum descriptive length principle. Calculated by using MDL. R function, MDL value achieves minimum when the number of compartments is 3.

3.2 Datasets

The software tool can be readily applied to various heterogeneous datasets. In the sample datasets, we provide three groups of data, including gene expression data, DCE-MRI image data and aerial image data to help users explore the potential use of the software tool. In the gene expression dataset, the raw measured gene expression data were generated by our collaborators at Georgetown University Medical School, where the mRNA was derived from MCF7 (cancer) and HS27 (stroma) cell lines, and then biologically mixed to obtain mixed mRNA expression profiles [23]. mRNA samples from two breast cancer cell lines were extracted and mixed at proportions designed to mimic actual biological tumor samples. Dynamic contrast-enhanced magnetic resonance imaging (DCE-MRI) provides a noninvasive in vivo method to evaluate tumor vasculature architectures based on contrast accumulation and washout [24]. In this dataset, the snapshots of DCE-MRI sequence are taken from the same tumor at 26 time points (Fig. 5a) [25]. The third dataset consists of mixtures of three natural images, each of which contains 103×103 pixels.

The processing steps in the Data preprocessing section need to be followed if readers are working on gene expression datasets.

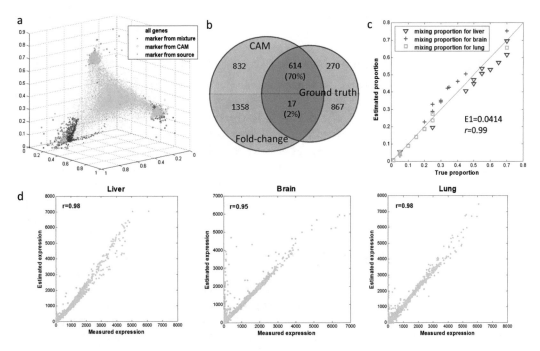

Fig. 6 Validation of CAM for blindly identifying subpopulation-specific marker genes (distinct subpopulations include liver, lung, and brain)

3.3 Anticipated Results

Here we discuss the anticipated results that can be achieved by executing this method to analyze gene expression data. This dataset, containing gene expression profiles from mixed rat liver, brain, and lung biospecimens, can be downloaded from GEO website through the access code GSE19830.

Unsupervised identification of marker genes from mixed expression data allows us to acquire the relative expression levels of those genes (Fig. 1a). The average of sum-normalized marker gene expressions produces subpopulation proportions (**Note 4** and Fig. 1b). Using predesigned RNA mixing experimental data acquired from biological mixtures of pure gene expressions (brain, liver, lung) [5, 6], we showed that CAM identified the marker genes that define each of the multiple subpopulations (Fig. 6a, b) and estimated the proportions of these subpopulations in the mixed samples (Fig. 6c) and their respective expression profiles (Fig. 6d).

Since the presence of marker genes is both a sufficient and necessary condition for deconvolution (**Note 4**), these results (validated by the ground truth) confirm the existence of marker genes and CAM's ability to detect these genes blindly and correctly (Fig. 6b). Moreover, CAM enabled detection of condition-specific marker genes across sample groups (for example, disease versus control). Thus, novel marker genes for a subpopulation in a given context can be determined, despite an expected change in that subpopulation's relative abundance and/or state.

4 Notes

1. Algorithms involved in each step.

   (a) Data preprocessing.

   First, we eliminate genes whose signal intensity (vector norm) is lower than 5% (noise) or higher than 95% (outlier) of the mean value over all genes. The signals from these genes are unreliable and could have a negative impact on the subsequent analyses. Second, when $J \gg K$, dimension reduction is performed on the raw measurements using principal component analysis, sample clustering or nonnegative matrix factorization techniques, to improve the efficiency of subsequent analyses [13, 26].

   (b) Gene expression clustering.

   To further improve the efficiency of CAM algorithm, we aggregate gene vectors into representative clusters using affinity propagation clustering (APC) [18, 19, 26, 30]. As an initialization-free and near-global-optimum clustering method, APC simultaneously considers all gene vectors as potential exemplars and recursively exchanges real-valued 'messages' between gene vectors until a high-quality set of exemplars and corresponding clusters gradually emerge. The APC algorithm is data-driven, so the message-passing procedure may be terminated after a fixed number of iterations or after the updates stay constant for some number of iterations. In all of our experiments, we adopted a default damping factor of 0.5. The update rules are repeated iteratively and terminated when no further change occurs for about 10 iterations [19, 26]. Our experience indicates that these default algorithmic parameter settings are quite suitable for obtaining good results.

   (c) Convex analysis of mixtures (CAM) algorithm.

   - Latent variable model on mixed gene expressions in heterogeneous samples.

     Consider gene expression measured from a sample composed of K subpopulations. We assume that the measured expression level x is the weighted sum of each subpopulation's expression, where the contribution from a single subpopulation is proportional to the abundance and specific expression of that subpopulation [2, 5, 6, 10, 16]. The measured expression level thus is (Fig. 1c).

$$x_j(i) = \sum_{k=1}^{K} a_{jk}s_k(i),\qquad(1)$$

where $s_k(i)$ is the expression level of gene i in subpopulation k, $x_j(i)$ is the expression level of gene i in heterogeneous sample j, and a_{jk} is the proportion of subpopulation k in heterogeneous sample j. We further assume that gene expression values are nonnegative (before log-transformation [13, 16]) and adopt the definition of subpopulation-specific marker genes as those genes whose expression values are exclusively enriched in a particular subpopulation [6, 10, 11] (Fig. 1a). Thus, the specific expression of a marker gene (MG) in subpopulation k^* is

$$s_{k*}(i_{\mathrm{MG}-k}) = \begin{cases} s_{k*}(i_{\mathrm{MG}-k}) > 0, & k = k^*; \\ 0, & k \neq k^*. \end{cases}\qquad(2)$$

When marker genes are known for each subpopulation, we can use the expression values of marker genes to deconvolve mixed expression profiles [6, 10, 11]. When no such prior knowledge is available (i.e., none of K, a_{jk} and $s_k(i_{\mathrm{MG}})$ is known *a priori*), solving latent variable model (Eq. 1) is essentially a blind source separation problem [21, 22], where accurate identification of subpopulation-specific marker genes is a critical but nontrivial task [6, 10, 27].

Our formulation dissects complex transcriptional heterogeneity into combinations of distinct subpopulations, leveraging the advantages of both tissue-wide and single-cell approaches [14, 28]. Specifically, discerning differences among single cells can gain valuable information about intercellular heterogeneity but allow only a few markers per cell and is prone to cell-cycle confounders; while tissue-wide measures provide a detailed picture of averaged population state but at the cost of losing information about intersubpopulation heterogeneity.

- Parallelism between latent variable model and the theory of convex sets.

  Consider a set of $J (\geq K)$ heterogeneous samples of varying composition of unknown subpopulations. Applying a sum-based standardization to gene expression values $x_j(i)$ across samples and using vector-matrix notation, we can reexpress Eq. 1 as

$$x(i) = \sum_{k=1}^{K} s_k(i) a_k \qquad (3)$$

where $x(i)$ and a_k are the vector notations (over samples) of mixed expression values and subpopulation proportions, respectively. Since $s_k(i)$ is nonnegative and standardized, as a nonnegative linear combination of $\{a_k\}$, the set of gene expression vectors $x(i)$ forms a subset of the *convex set* uniquely defined by the set of $\{a_k\}$ [18, 21, 29] (Fig. 1b)

$$X = \left\{ \sum_{k=1}^{K} s_k(i) a_k, s_k(i) \geq 0, \sum_{k=1}^{K} s_k(i) = 1, i = 1, \ldots, N \right\} \qquad (4)$$

where N is the number of genes.

- Mathematical foundation for unsupervised identification of novel marker genes.

  We propose the convex analysis of mixtures (CAM) framework to exploit the strong parallelism between a linear latent variable model (Eq. 3) and the theory of convex sets. The novel insight is that subpopulation-specific marker genes that define pure subpopulations reside at the extremities of the scatter simplex formed by all genes, while the interior of the simplex is occupied by coexpressed genes (whose values are linear nonnegative combinations of pure subpopulation expression values) (Fig. 1b). We can then identify novel marker genes by geometrically locating the vertices of the multifaceted simplex that most tightly encloses the gene expression profiles and has the same number of subpopulations as vertices. CAM is supported theoretically by a well-grounded mathematical framework as summarized in the following newly proven theorems.

Lemma 1 (Scatter Compression and Rotation): Suppose that pure subpopulation expressions are nonnegative, and $x(i) = a_1 s_1(i) + \ldots + a_k s_k(i) + \ldots + a_K s_K(i)$ where a_k's are linearly independent and nonnegative, then, the scatter simplex of pure subpopulation expressions is compressed and rotated to form the scatter simplex of mixed expressions whose vertices coincide with a_k's.

Theorem 1 (Unsupervised Identifiability): Suppose that pure subpopulation expressions are nonnegative and subpopulation-specific marker genes exist for each constituting subpopulation, and $x(i) = a_1 s_1(i) + \ldots + a_k s_k(i) + \ldots + a_K s_K(i)$ where a_k's are linearly independent, then, the vertices of the scatter simplex of mixed expressions host subpopulation-specific marker genes and coincide with $\boldsymbol{a}_k$'s that can be readily estimated from marker gene expression values with appropriate rescaling.

From Lemma 1 and Theorem 1, there is a feasible mathematical solution to identify subpopulation-specific marker genes directly from the measured gene expression mixtures: in principle, under a noise-free scenario, we can blindly identify novel marker gene indices by locating the vertices of the mixed expression scatter simplex [19, 22, 26]. We emphasize that CAM can distinguish between phenotypically similar subpopulations, by working in scatter space in which the power of detecting simplex vertices depends solely on the mixture diversity (a basic requirement for any inverse problem) rather than phenotypic diversity [14].

To identify the vertices of clustered scatter simplex of mixed expression profiles X, on the M cluster centers $\{\boldsymbol{g}_m\}$, we assumed K true vertices and conducted an exhaustive combinatorial search (with total C_K^M combinations), based on a convex-hull-to-data fitting criterion, to identify the most probable K vertices. We used the margin-of-error

$$\delta_{m,\{1,...K\}\in C_K^M} = \min_{\alpha_1,...\alpha_K} \left\| \boldsymbol{g}_m - \sum_{k=1}^{K} \alpha_k \boldsymbol{g}_k \right\|_2,$$
$$\alpha_k \geq 0, \sum_{k=1}^{K} \alpha_k = 1, \tag{5}$$

to quantify the 'mismatch' between $\boldsymbol{g}_m$ and convex set X defined by $\{\boldsymbol{g}_k = 1, ..., K\}$, where we have $\delta_{m,\{1,...K\}\in C_K^M} = 0$ if $\boldsymbol{g}_m$ is inside X. We then selected the most probable K vertices when the corresponding sum of the margin-of-error between the convex hull and the remaining "exterior" cluster centers reaches its minimum [18, 22, 26]:

$$\{\boldsymbol{g}_{k=1^*,...,K^*}\} = \operatorname*{argmin}_{\{1,...K\}\in C_K^M} \sum_{m=1}^{M} \delta_{m,\{1,...K\}\in C_K^M} \tag{6}$$

Subsequently, we identified the indices of subpopulation-specific marker genes based on the memberships associated with $\{\boldsymbol{g}_{k=1}^*, ..., K^*\}$, where $\{1^*, ..., K^*\}$ denote the cluster indices of the true simplex vertices, and the genes assigned to gene cluster at a vertex $\{i|i \in \boldsymbol{g}_k^*\}$ are declared to be marker genes, i.e., $\mathrm{MG}_k = \{i|i \in \boldsymbol{g}_k^*\}$.

2. Estimation of the proportions and specific expression profiles of subpopulations.

On the basis of the expression levels of subpopulation-specific marker genes detected by CAM, the relative proportions of constituent subpopulations are estimated using standardized averaging,

$$\widehat{a}_k = \frac{1}{n_{\text{MG}-k}} \sum_{i \in \text{MG}-k} \frac{x(i)}{\|x(i)\|}, k = 1, \ldots K, \tag{7}$$

where MG-k is the index set of marker genes for subpopulation k; $n_{\text{MG}-k}$ is the number of marker genes for subpopulation k; and $\|.\|$ denotes the vector norm (L_1 or L_2). The resulting $\{\widehat{a}_k\}$ are then used to deconvolve the mixed expressions into subpopulation-specific profiles by nonnegative least-square regression techniques [6, 10, 11, 18, 26].

3. Model selection procedure.

One important discovery step for CAM (as a fully unsupervised method) is to automatically detect the number K of cell subpopulations in the heterogeneous samples. We used MDL, a widely adopted and consistent information theoretic criterion [17], to guide model selection [18]. We performed CAM on several competing candidates, and selected the optimal model that assigns high probabilities to the observed data with parameters that are not too complex to encode [17]. Specifically, a model is selected with K subpopulations by minimizing the total description code length defined by [18]

$$\text{MDL}(K) = -\log(\mathcal{L}(X_M|\theta(K))) + \frac{(K-1)J}{2}\log(M)$$
$$+ \frac{KM}{2}\log(J), \tag{8}$$

where $\mathcal{L}(\cdot)$ denotes the joint likelihood function of the clustered latent variable model, X_M denotes the set of M gene vector cluster centers, and $\theta(K)$ denotes the set of freely adjustable parameters in the clustered latent variable model [18, 19, 26].

4. When you double-click CAM-Java.jar and there is no dialog showing up, please make sure you followed all the steps in Subheading 2. The R and Java environments have to be correctly installed beforehand. If you use Ubuntu operating system, you may not open the software by double-clicking without modifying the system properties. Instead you can open it by typing "*java -jar CAM-Java.jar*" in the terminal under the path of the software.

5. After successfully loading the data, there might be some error information dialog popping up when clicking the 'run' button. The most possible reason is that Runiversal or R.matlab

packages are not installed correctly. You need to install these two packages manually beforehand. Another possible reason is that when you use the test dataset, you did not select the right corresponding algorithm for the data. For example, you should apply CAM-ICA to datasets in data_correlation folder, CAM-CM to data_DCE_MRI, and CAM-nWCA to data_ image. If the above scenarios do not apply to your case, please check the Application status bar carefully and follow the instructions.

In general, the detailed information in Application status bar will tell you how to resolve the problem. Most errors are due to missing necessary packages or loading the wrong dataset.

6. The time required to run this software tool is mainly related to the size of the dataset and CPU power. The complete procedure usually takes less than 10 min for each of the three sample datasets.

References

1. Hoffman EP, Awad T, Palma J, Webster T, Hubbell E, Warrington JA, Spira A, Wright GW, Buckley J, Triche T, Davis R, Tibshirani R, Xiao W, Jones W, Tompkins R, West M (2004) Expression profiling-best practices for data generation and interpretation in clinical trials. Nat Rev Genet 5:229–237

2. Stuart RO, Wachsman W, Berry CC, Wang J, Wasserman L, Klacansky I, Masys D, Arden K, Goodison S, McClellend M, Wang Y, Sawyers A, Kalcheva I, Tarin D, Mercola D (2004) In silico dissection of cell-type-associated patterns of gene expression in prostate cancer. Proc Natl Acad Sci U S A 101 (2):615–620

3. Junttila MR, de Sauvage FJ (2013) Influence of tumour micro-environment heterogeneity on therapeutic response. Nature 501 (7467):346–354

4. Kreso A, O'Brien CA, van Galen P, Gan OI, Notta F, Brown AM, Ng K, Ma J, Wienholds E, Dunant C, Pollett A, Gallinger S, McPherson J, Mulligan CG, Shibata D, Dick JE (2013) Variable clonal repopulation dynamics influence chemotherapy response in colorectal cancer. Science 339 (6119):543–548

5. Shen-Orr SS, Tibshirani R, Khatri P, Bodian DL, Staedtler F, Perry NM, Hastie T, Sarwal MM, Davis MM, Butte AJ (2010) Cell type-specific gene expression differences in complex tissues. Nat Methods 7(4):287–289

6. Kuhn A, Thu D, Waldvogel HJ, Faull RL, Luthi-Carter R (2011) Population-specific expression analysis (PSEA) reveals molecular changes in diseased brain. Nat Methods 8 (11):945–947

7. Yu G, Li H, Ha S, Shih Ie M, Clarke R, Hoffman EP, Madhavan S, Xuan J, Wang Y (2011) PUGSVM: a caBIG analytical tool for multiclass gene selection and predictive classification. Bioinformatics 27(5):736–738

8. Shapiro E, Biezuner T, Linnarsson S (2013) Single-cell sequencing-based technologies will revolutionize whole-organism science. Nat Rev Genet 14(9):618–630

9. Yuan Y, Failmezger H, Rueda OM, Ali HR, Graf S, Chin SF, Schwarz RF, Curtis C, Dunning MJ, Bardwell H, Johnson N, Doyle S, Turashvili G, Provenzano E, Aparicio S, Caldas C, Markowetz F (2012) Quantitative image analysis of cellular heterogeneity in breast tumors complements genomic profiling. Sci Transl Med 4(157):157ra143

10. Lu P, Nakorchevskiy A, Marcotte EM (2003) Expression deconvolution: a reinterpretation of DNA microarray data reveals dynamic changes in cell populations. Proc Natl Acad Sci U S A 100(18):10370–10375

11. Abbas AR, Wolslegel K, Seshasayee D, Modrusan Z, Clark HF (2009) Deconvolution of blood microarray data identifies cellular activation patterns in systemic lupus erythematosus. PLoS One 4(7):e6098

12. Zuckerman NS, Noam Y, Goldsmith AJ, Lee PP (2013) A self-directed method for cell-type identification and separation of gene expression microarrays. PLoS Comput Biol 9(8): e1003189

13. Gaujoux R, Seoighe C (2012) Semi-supervised nonnegative matrix factorization for gene expression deconvolution: a case study. Infect Genet Evol 12(5):913–921

14. Schwartz R, Shackney SE (2010) Applying unmixing to gene expression data for tumor phylogeny inference. BMC Bioinformatics 11:42

15. Hart Y, Sheftel H, Hausser J, Szekely P, Ben-Moshe NB, Korem Y, Tendler A, Mayo AE, Alon U (2015) Inferring biological tasks using Pareto analysis of high-dimensional data. Nat Methods 12(3):233–235

16. Zhong Y, Liu Z (2012) Gene expression deconvolution in linear space. Nat Methods 9 (1):8–9. Author reply 9

17. Wax M, Kailath T (1985) Detection of signals by information theoretic criteria. IEEE Trans Acoustics Speech Signal Process 33 (2):387–392

18. Chen L, Choyke PL, Chan TH, Chi CY, Wang G, Wang Y (2011) Tissue-specific compartmental analysis for dynamic contrast-enhanced MR imaging of complex tumors. IEEE Trans Med Imaging 30(12):2044–2058

19. Chen L, Chan TH, Choyke PL, Hillman EM, Chi CY, Bhujwalla ZM, Wang G, Wang SS, Szabo Z, Wang Y (2011) CAM-CM: a signal deconvolution tool for in vivo dynamic contrast-enhanced imaging of complex tissues. Bioinformatics 27(18):2607–2609

20. Oja E, Plumbley M (2004) Blind separation of positive sources by globally convergent gradient search. Neural Comput 16:1811–1825

21. Chan TH, Ma WK, Chi CY, Wang Y (2008) A convex analysis framework for blind separation of non-negative sources. IEEE Trans Signal Process 56(10):5120–5134

22. Wang FY, Chi CY, Chan TH, Wang Y (2010) Nonnegative least-correlated component analysis for separation of dependent sources by volume maximization. IEEE Trans Pattern Anal Mach Intell 32(5):875–888

23. Wang N, Gong T, Clarke R, Chen L, Shih Ie M, Zhang Z, Levine DA, Xuan J, Wang Y (2015) UNDO: a Bioconductor R package for unsupervised deconvolution of mixed gene expressions in tumor samples. Bioinformatics 31(1):137–139

24. McDonald DM, Choyke PL (2003) Imaging of angiogenesis: from microscope to clinic. Nat Med 9:713–725

25. Chen L, Choyke PL, Wang N, Clarke R, Bhujwalla ZM, Hillman EM, Wang G, Wang Y (2014) Unsupervised deconvolution of dynamic imaging reveals intratumor vascular heterogeneity and repopulation dynamics. PLoS One 9(11):e112143

26. Wang N, Meng F, Chen L, Madhavan S, Clarke R, Hoffman E-P, Xuan J, Wang Y (2013) The CAM software for nonnegative blind source separation in R-Java. J Mach Learn Res 14:2899–2903

27. Kuhn A, Kumar A, Beilina A, Dillman A, Cookson MR, Singleton AB (2012) Cell population-specific expression analysis of human cerebellum. BMC Genomics 13:610

28. Buettner F, Natarajan KN, Casale FP, Proserpio V, Scialdone A, Theis FJ, Teichmann SA, Marioni JC, Stegle O (2015) Computational analysis of cell-to-cell heterogeneity in single-cell RNA-sequencing data reveals hidden subpopulations of cells. Nat Biotechnol 33(2):155–160

29. Boyd S, Vandenberghe L (2004) Convex optimization, 1st edn. Cambridge University Press, Cambridge

30. Frey BJ, Dueck D (2007) Clustering by Passing Messages Between Data Points. Science 315 (5814):972–976

INDEX

A

Alternative splicing (AS) 73, 78, 80, 82, 84, 202

B

Bioconductor...7, 18–22, 24,
    28, 29, 36, 37, 45, 46, 50, 52, 111, 118, 119, 127,
    129, 210
Blind source separation 231

C

Cell type................................ 73, 139, 209, 210, 212–220
CLIP-seq, *see* Small RNAs
Clustering 27, 32, 80, 121,
    129, 130, 132, 133, 210, 211, 213–215, 218,
    228, 230
Convex analysis of mixture (CAM)............ 224, 230, 232
CPAT 140, 146, 147, 149
CsrA 171–173
Cufflinks..6, 9, 13, 74,
    140, 144, 146, 147, 149, 218

D

Data deconvolution 229
De novo transcriptome assembly....................................4, 8
DESeq.. 7–9, 15,
    43, 155, 160, 161
Differential expression 7, 9, 13,
    18, 24, 25, 49, 50, 110, 119, 129, 140, 144, 147,
    149, 155, 159–161, 210, 218
Directional RNA-Seq...90–92, 98
Driving force 210, 217, 220

F

Feature selection 191, 193

G

Gene expression analysis 8–14, 24, 27, 155, 174
Gene expression variation 183–196
Gene set enrichment analysis (GSEA) 28,
    36, 38–42, 134, 135, 179, 180
Genefilter 23
Genomic imprinting 199

H

Hfq 171–173, 178

I

Intrinsic noise 183

L

Limma................................... 24, 26, 32, 52, 128–130, 132
Long intergenic noncoding RNAs (lincRNAs,
    lncRNAs) 139–149
Long-read sequencing, *see* PacBio sequencing

M

Machine learning............... 184, 185, 187, 191, 193, 196
Marker genes 212, 214,
    215, 219, 223–225, 229, 231–234
Maternal and paternal contributions 200,
    202, 203, 207
Microarray 3, 17–20,
    22–24, 29, 37, 48, 127–135, 185, 191
Microarray data analysis 17–32, 128, 185
MicroRNAs (miRNAs) 109–114,
    116, 118–122, 124, 127, 128, 132–135, 139
mirPRo 110, 111, 113, 116, 117

N

Network.. 35, 129,
    132, 134, 135, 184, 193, 210, 217, 220
Next-generation sequencing (NGS) 3, 7, 154, 209
NGS data analysis..209
Noncoding RNA (ncRNA) 83, 97,
    139, 140, 171
Non-model organism...3, 4, 8, 9
Normalization 18–20, 23,
    29, 121, 129, 130, 160, 210, 212, 213, 218

O

Operon 90, 92

P

PacBio sequencing 75, 85
Pathway.................................. 28, 35, 127, 134, 174, 218

Pipeline 19, 58, 75, 76,
    90, 92, 98, 104, 110, 113, 116, 117, 128, 132,
    173, 174, 201–203, 210, 212, 234
Posttranscriptional modification 101
ProQ 171, 172

Q

QuickRNASeq 57–69

R

R package 9, 18, 19, 23,
    27, 36–39, 43, 46, 48, 62, 111, 118, 128, 129,
    132, 134, 135, 180, 204, 210
RIP-seq, *see* Small RNAs
RNA editing 101–107
RNA sequencing (RNA-Seq) 75, 202

S

Signature gene 215–217
Single-cell RNA-Seq 140, 210
Single cells 140, 184, 193,
    196, 200, 209–220, 231
Small RNA sequencing 109
Small RNAs (sRNAs) 92, 158, 178
SpliceHunter, *see* Alternative splicing

STAR 58–60, 62,
    140, 141, 143, 144, 147, 155, 156, 158–160, 164
Support vector regression (SVR) 184,
    187–190, 192–196

T

TEtranscripts 153–166
Time course analysis 73
Tissue heterogeneity 223, 224
Topology 35, 36, 43–51
Transcript border
    start site 90, 94, 95
    termination site 90, 94
    unit 77, 81, 90–93
Transcript isoform, *see* Alternative splicing
Transcriptome 3, 4, 8,
    17, 35, 58, 74, 75, 89–91, 103, 130, 132, 133,
    144, 147, 155, 156, 174, 185, 200, 209
Transposable elements, *see* TEtranscripts

V

Visualization 19, 36, 42,
    58, 75–77, 80, 85, 129, 134, 174, 178, 179, 210,
    218

Printed in the United States
By Bookmasters